Drama Momma
in
the Land of UN

GWEN THORNE

Editing & Interior Design
Preserving the Author's Voice
www.ravendodd.com

Cover Image
Jackie Pecora
J. Pecora Creative Marketing Studio

Cover Layout
Design Consultant: Jennifer Smith

ISBN: 978-1-947678-15-6
Library of Congress Control Number: 2020902033

Published through:
Preserving the Author's Voice

Dedication

To all survivors and their families,
may you find peace in your hearts.

"rejoicing in hope; patient in tribulation;
continuing stedfastly in prayer"

(Rom. 12:12 ASV).

Acknowledgments

So many people helped make this book a reality. First, I want to thank the Lisa Foundation for believing in me and offering help and support in bringing this book to fruition. Especially Joan Kaplan, who is a Lisa Foundation board member who went above and beyond to encourage me to persevere.

I want to thank my family for putting up with me when I went into "writing-mode" and tuned everyone out.

Thank you to my editor, Raven Dodd, who patiently guided me through the tedious book birthing process.

Thank you to the CaringBridge website that enabled us to keep our friends and family updated on Jess's journey. We were able to stay in constant communication with messages of hope, love, prayers, and support. The CaringBridge community was a real blessing during a most challenging time.

Finally, I want to thank Jess for teaching me to see the world anew and reminding me that every day is full of bunches of sunshine.

Foreword

As a developer helping Todd Crawford, husband of Lisa Colagrossi and the Founder of The Lisa Foundation, I met Gwen Thorne and her daughter at a luncheon for Southwest Florida brain aneurysm survivors.

Although supported by a Lee County group at the time, they were looking for additional backing and invited us to meet with them. We had a second meeting with even more survivors and their caregivers at Lois Colagrossi's home. Lois is the mother of Lisa Colagrossi, who was an ABC TV NY Anchor who died suddenly of a brain aneurysm on her way home from a news assignment. This news reverberated around the globe. The Lisa Foundation was started to help educate and make people aware of brain aneurysms, the symptoms, and prevention.

It was obvious to me that Gwen and her daughter Jessica were extraordinary people with the will and determination to improve Jessica's lot in life after she survived a brain aneurysm. The story of her extremely hard work to walk, talk, and be a contributing member of society again is astounding.

My more than 32 years' experience on the Greater New England Board of MS taught me that nothing is impossible. I could help the Foundation and educate many people that you can achieve your goals through the story of Gwen and Jessica.

Gwen told me she wrote a book, which I read. As the Chair of a Book Club with over 75 members, I am familiar with writing styles as well as descriptive information. Her writing style is impressive. The facts are so compelling and can help countless other survivors who tell similar stories. Gwen's sense of humor also sheds some fun on such a serious subject.

Jessica can now walk, talk, swim, and do so many things she could not do prior to her help from Gwen and her dad. I am so proud of all of them.

As a result, I became a Member of the Board of The Lisa Foundation and do fundraising, connect people with the right doctors, work with people in the medical device business, and contribute to what has become known as the best charitable brain aneurysm Foundation in the country.

Gwen is donating 10% of her proceeds to The Lisa Foundation. I think this is a book you cannot put down.

Joan Kaplan
lisafoundation.org

Introduction

What inspires people to write? Life is our storyteller. It's undeniable. It's the human experience with the gamut of emotions; joy, love, sorrow, sadness, even deeper—unfathomable.

Often, I struggle to find words to express the depths of my emotions. Some authors strive to make a story unforgettable by enhancing the narrative with extraordinary characters or situations that tease the imagination. In this case, the narrative is true. There is not a drop of fiction in it. It is also strange. I wish it were fiction. It is about my life in the Land of UN.

Drama Momma in the Land of UN came to me in the middle of the night as I struggled with the sleep-deprived thoughts rattling my brain. The Drama Momma part was easy. I am, after all, a first-class card-carrying drama momma. As the hours slowed to a steady drip, drip, drip of minutes, I stared at the ceiling UNblinking, UNmoving, UNable to sleep and trying desperately to UNthink my clambering thoughts. Then, I realized this is me. I'm surrounded by "UNs!" I live in the Land of UN.

Not having the luxury of waiting to spill my thoughts on paper lest I forget them, I groggily meandered to my keyboard. In my case, the writing spirit moves me mostly between midnight and 4 a.m.

So, at three o'clock in the morning, my fingers pecked holes in the silent stillness typing non-stop in the shadowy pre-dawn Land of UN. It's been a labor of love, weaving the events, and trying to sew words together to present an accurate picture.

If this story were a patchwork quilt, the patches might appear to be helter-skelter. Once put together, though, the quilt tells the story of a lifetime. My lifetime. I am Gwen. My quilt seems simple enough at a glance, but it's not. This story contains a lot of drama with some interesting characters. You will notice that I give certain characters unflattering nicknames. This was my perception at the time and does not necessarily reflect how I feel now.

There are many patches that I believe most people will relate to and understand. Then again, there are many patches that no one will understand because it is impossible to fathom the depths of despair that birthed this book.

Despair is only one part of the story. I'd like to think that the rest of the story is full of hope, joy, and love. I hope that the words I've sewn together will draw the reader into my Land of UN and that they may even see themselves in it.

In this land, some unthinkable things happen. It's an uncanny land of real-life struggles and real-life joy. When you enter it, hopefully, you will emerge unscathed but not untouched.

Let the quilting begin...

Chapter 1

UNkempt

The Farm

December 2016

Something in the air caught my attention as I strolled through the shade, clutching my laptop. Instead of searching for a log on which to sit, I went in search of the smell. I stood for a moment under the towering oak trees in the hopes that the shade would cool the hot, humid air. I was wrong. The familiar smell was adding to the thick swelter. It wasn't a pleasant smell like flowers or anything green and pretty.

It didn't smell pretty. It smelled dirty... and unkempt. Did I smell homeless? No. Not homeless. Almost, though. I remember smelling homeless behind the park where I used to work. I knew that smell, and this wasn't it. This smell awoke a distant memory in the recesses of my brain. Long ago, I smelled this when I was walking in the hundred acres behind my house. It intrigued me then, and it intrigued me now.

It didn't take long to find the smell's origin tucked under a fallen limb where I would not sit—not today anyway. There, blending with the shades of brown, was an indiscernible shifting shape. But for the smell, I would not have noticed the four or five piglets huddled together. I guessed they were less than a week old, which meant that the momma pig had to be close by.

Piglets didn't scare me, but wild momma pigs did. I quickly made my retreat to a distance I felt was safe enough and found a less threatening branch on which to unwind and write.

I figured it might take me a while to relax, so I needed a comfortable spot. Was there such a thing as a soft branch? No, but I had enough padding to endure sitting for at least an hour. An hour away from the house was more than enough time to mull over the thoughts ricocheting through my brain. I had given up on writing for a long time. Was an hour long enough, or did I need days—weeks maybe?

It was hot as if the trees were holding their breath, adding to the heat. Nothing moved; not even the piglets made a sound. Strange. I don't know if piglets are noisy, but I expected to hear some grunting coming from the piglet lair. I was sure I'd hear them when their mom returned.

So, there I sat on the less menacing branch. Waiting. I didn't know what I was waiting for. Was I expecting a burning bush or perhaps a ray of brilliant sunshine illuminating an angel? As if on cue, a perfect circle of light appeared on the ground in front of me. No aberration accompanied the sunlight, and no voice spoke to me. It just glimmered there taunting my imagination to make something of the luminescence. *Perhaps I should fabricate a divine messenger heralding great promise*, I thought. *Maybe, if I step into the light, I'll be baptized with great wisdom and will write something wise and inspiring.*

I step into the light. It's hot. I go back to my log in the shade. For a moment, I sit toad-like with my laptop perched on the branch by my side. *What did I come to write—to ponder?* I wonder. *My life?* 58 years to be exact.

Today is my birthday. It's December in Florida, and it's hot. It doesn't feel like Christmas time. It doesn't feel like my birthday. A December birthday right after Christmas was always a bit of a disappointment when I was growing up because the "combined presents" were inevitable.

I never really understood the combined presents. One year I got a unicycle—my only request for Christmas. My dad informed me that the unicycle was a combined Christmas/birthday present. So, naturally, I wondered why I didn't just get the wheel on Christmas and the rest of the unicycle on my birthday.

I taught myself how to ride the unicycle by holding onto the walls in the house. By the time I became a one-wheeled pro, every wall was as nicked and bruised as my shins and knees. The unicycle seat and pedals left permanent gouges in the wood floors throughout the hallways. When the handprints outnumbered the flowers on the wallpaper, I was banished from the house and graduated to riding between the cars in the driveway. I know the vehicles took a unicycle beating too, so I was given the ultimatum to either master the art of unicycling without props or give it up.

I never give up! So, after months of daily unicycle battles, I finally won the fight and took my first tentative no-props ride down the driveway. Within six months, I was riding backward, going up and down steps, playing basketball, and carrying my three sisters (one on each leg and one on my shoulders) all while riding my unicycle. It was as if the unicycle became an extension of my body. I was rarely without it and often rode to the store a mile away. I always had my hamster, Snowball, in my pocket while I rode. It's a wonder he survived.

The unicycle did come in handy a few years back when I was "Skiddles," the sweetest clown in town. I still rode that unicycle like a pro! I raced kids holding rubber chickens and did wheelies around the bases at home baseball games for our local team. I was a great clown until my knees killed my unicycle escapades, and my fingers protested balloon tying. It was good money, but I had to face the reality that Skiddles, the clown, had finally grown too old for her unicycle. The unicycle is tucked away in the corner of the garage now, waiting for another clown to rescue it.

Unicycles, clowns, and combined childhood presents are all in the past now. I didn't come out here to mull over those things. I didn't come out here to ponder my birthday. I didn't come out here to reflect on birthday presents or lack thereof. What did I come out here for? I guess I came to find God. I came out here to ask God to inspire my writing.

Lately, God has been hiding from me. He's been chiding me with His absence or lack of availability. I don't know. I don't know much of anything these days. Is He absent from my life or just not available? Is it Him or me? Am I the one leaving God out of my life? My life... I can't finish the sentence. Why is it just "my life"? I mean, there are so many other lives crisscrossed in this one life, like a big ball of twine.

Here I sit in the swelter of an unusually warm December day in Florida. I wonder, am I able to tell a story that keeps you on the edge of your seat? I'm on the edge of my log now. My butt hurts, and my knees creak. My brain dissolves—evaporates into the dryness. The dryness is in my fingers, too. No story right now in this dryness. Not today.

Maybe it was a story back then. Perhaps it was a story worth telling once upon a time. I don't know that it's a story worth telling now. People ask me to tell it. They say, "You should write a book." Or, "Your life is like a book." Or, "You were on Oprah!" So what. So what if I was on Oprah? So what if my life is book material? I'm sure there are lots of lives out there that are book-worthy. Why me? Why my life?

Someone once called me a "drama momma" because my life is so full of drama all the time. I don't think he meant it to be complimentary, but I kind of like the title of Drama Momma. It suits me. I'm a drama momma now, but the drama started in 1960 when my mother died. I hadn't even reached toddlerhood yet.

Fragments. That's what I'm made of. Tragic fragments..."tragments." Three children left behind with a dad that didn't know what to do with his broken life. I keep thinking of broken glass—shards and slivers everywhere—tragments. Impossible to glue back together, so you do the best you can to reconstruct the shatters. You make something that resembles the old, but tragments cannot be put back together again because mommies don't just reappear out of nowhere. Putting tragments back together again is like trying to glue Humpty Dumpty together again.

That was what my dad tried to do. He called all the king's horses and all the king's men. In this case, he called all the grandmas and aunts, but they couldn't—they just couldn't. Shattered lives. Tragments. That's what I remember.

The tragments were glued, epoxied, and cemented. I and my brother and sister were glued together, and we survived as kids will do. I even grew up despite my rebellious stage that involved drinking my way into oblivion. Oblivion was good back then. I was about thirteen-years-old when I had my first drink. I don't know how or why I had so much access to alcohol, but I know I drank a lot for a long time.

Whiskey, beer, and moonshine erasers were my constant companions. They took me places I wanted to be—mostly nowhere. They took me to nowhere and back—then back to nowhere again. I don't know when I left nowhere, but I think it was when I was about twenty-five. Maybe, if I were brutally honest, I'd say nowhere isn't far behind me. It's a place I've become all too familiar with over time.

Did I mention it's my birthday? I thought that I'd become wise with age. What I've discovered is that I've become old as the years have progressed. That's it—just old. Old and perhaps a bit crankier.

The pigs are noisy now. Maybe Momma has found her way back. I'd go see, but I don't wish to disturb a mother boar and her piglets, nor do I wish to see if the daddy boar is close by. Out of the corner of my eye, I spot Felix. "Hey Felix," I yell as if he'll answer me. He looks my way, snorts his response, and gallops through the trees, leaving dust clouds in his wake.

Maybe it was Felix who disturbed the pigs. Perhaps it was Fred who is now visible in the clearing. Felix is lucky to have Fred as his constant companion. I wonder if they communicate with each other—dog to horse. I decide they must. Otherwise, why stay so close to each other?

"Are you God?" I ask the sunny spot that lights up the ground in front of me. No answer. "Of course, you are," I say to the spot. "You're God. The trees are God. Felix is God. All of you are God in one way or the other, aren't you?" *I'm so wise,* I think to myself. *I see God in everything.* "So, God," I'm yelling now at the spot. "Why did you let this happen to my daughter?!"

It wasn't a question that I expected an answer to. I've learned that God doesn't answer questions through sunny spots on the ground. My anger flares as bright as the perfect circular light in front of me. It flares in my soul. So much anger. Yet, I feel strangely calm. I am an oxymoron. Or maybe I'm just a moron.

On the outside, I'm the perfect Christian woman saying all the right things about my daughter's tragedy—God's will and all that jazz. On the inside, I'm a raving lunatic. Rage is not the right word for what my gut feels. Rage is too mild—milquetoast. What's the word? Indignation? No. Mania? No. Rampage? No. Rampageous? No. No word is adequate. No word will tell the truth about what I feel right now as I stare at the God spot in front of me. I have no words with which to spin this yarn.

Chapter 2

UNfolding

Day 1

October 27, 2015

My beautiful daughter Jessica has suffered a brain aneurysm. I could spend this time updating her medical condition, but that does not define Jessica. This is what defines Jessica: "Strength and dignity are her clothing..." (Prov. 31:25). I asked God to give me a sign that my baby would be well and whole again. I went to the chapel, and I opened the bible right to Jessica's favorite passage.

In its entirety, the passage describes everything that is Jess: "A worthy woman who can find? For her price is far above rubies...She riseth also while it is yet night, And giveth food to her household...She stretcheth out her hand to the poor; Yea, she reacheth forth her hands to the needy" (Prov. 31:10, 15, 20).

I looked at Jess, who was hooked up to 27 IV bags. The ventilator was breathing for her. She was in a coma and was being kept comatose with a drug concoction that included fentanyl. She was completely unresponsive to any stimulation. Doctors were essentially keeping her alive for 24 hours to determine if there was any brain activity. Seizures, stroke, three surgeries by the second day, and her head shaved. A definite reality check!

However, my daughter will not be defined by a brain aneurysm. Yes, she is very, very sick right now, but she is better today than yesterday. Yes, she will have a long battle ahead, but amazingly powerful, godly people surround her, and she is so very strong. This is a journey of faith, hope, and love. And the greatest of these is love.

The Farm

December 2016

My mother died at the age of 32 in October 1960. It's uncanny the resemblance between what happened to my mother and what happened to Jess. What happened to both of them was horrific. Both my mother and Jess were young mothers with bright futures ahead of them. My mother had three children. Jess had one child, Eva, who was just three when the horror happened to Jess.

I call it horror because I don't know what else to call it. I was told by my daddy that my mother went to the store. Eva was told by her daddy that her mother had a boo-boo. Aaron, Eva's dad, didn't even call it a bad boo-boo! Both Eva and I were locked in the limbo of uncertainty.

Eva's mommy had to go to the hospital so the doctors could fix the boo-boo. That's it. In Eva's world, a boo-boo took her mommy away for more than three months, and nobody explained it to her.

In my 2-year-old world, my mommy was gone, but she wasn't coming back from the store. I wish someone had told me that Mommy wasn't coming back from the store. Maybe I wouldn't still be waiting for her to return. Perhaps I wouldn't get that weird empty feeling in the pit of my stomach every time someone tells me they're just running to the store on an errand. What store did

Mommy go to? The dead mommy store? Why do mommies go to the store and never come back?

The country song lyrics from "What Kinda Gone" start swimming in my head. I think it goes something like this: There's gone for good... gone with a long before it... Gone with the wind... I don't know. I do know that the song refers to all the good things that ain't never coming back. Sometimes I feel like chanting the words from Scarlet O'Hara in Gone with the Wind, "After all, tomorrow is another day."

What will tomorrow bring back? All the good things like a '59 Cadillac? No, probably not. I know it won't bring back dead mommies. Will it bring back Eva's mommy fully restored? No, it won't. Frankly, I just don't know what kinda gone we're talking about here.

Reflection

Recently, when my father passed away, I got some boxes from his house that I had not opened. When we moved, I opened one of the boxes and found a small carved box with many photos of my parents together before they were married. I always assumed that my father erased my mother from our lives and his life after my mother's death. This little memory box made me realize that he held onto her in his quiet way. It was hard for me to picture him reminiscing over the past as he wasn't an emotional man, but this box shed a whole new light on my father.

Now, I imagined him grieving over their lost life together. I could almost see and feel his tears, and it made me think how hard it must have been for him to face the world alone with three children to raise. He must have been terrified! I pictured him as a man overwhelmed with sadness and full of desperation.

He and my mother looked so happy together—so in love. I don't think I ever thought of them that way. I guess telling me that my mommy went to the store was my dad's way of protecting me from the overwhelming grief that he was feeling. Seeing these photos made me look at my father in a different light, and I realized that he was just doing what he felt was best for his kids.

Day 3

October 29, 2015

On the morning of Day 3, Jess went for another CT scan to determine if they could wake her up just a tiny bit. We were very hopeful about this development, and I thought of something that made me smile. Eva drew me a picture a few months before. When she handed it to me, she told me that it was full of bunches of sunshine for me.

The night before, my friend Lisa heard the song, "Glorious Unfolding" twice on the radio. She posted it to my Facebook page because it described Jess to a T. The second time it played on the radio, a rainbow appeared over the hospital. I took that as a sign of God's grace and promise. Jess had surgery to relieve the pressure in her head. She did well and was resting comfortably. The song "Glorious Unfolding" talks about a wonderful journey. This was Jess's wonderful journey. She was so strong and so loved. Maybe this was God's way of coming out of hiding.

Day 5

October 31, 2015

On Day 5, I took some deep breaths as I watched Jess. She was resting quietly. She had some of her skull removed the previous night to relieve the swelling of her brain. They told us they might start waking her up a bit, little by little, so we were just waiting to see how she reacted. Most of her head was shaved, but on a light-hearted note, she still had her braid.

Day 6

November 1, 2015

I know how frustrating and difficult it was for everyone waiting for updates on Jessica. I wish I could have given these updates with more certainty, but I just couldn't. We were waiting too. I was waiting for her smile, waiting to hear her beautiful voice, waiting for my baby to come back to me. What we did know is that the doctors were going to start waking her up very slowly to assess her. Taking the portion of her skull off had allowed her brain the ability to swell, which was a good thing. Essentially, no news at that time was good news. We were in this for the long haul, a minimum of 21 days in the ICU.

I cannot stress enough how amazing this hospital staff was. I know that the entire hospital prayed for her. The outpouring of support for our family was and still is nonstop. Every day, the ICU waiting room filled up with people from Jess's church, our church, co-workers, friends, and family. It was truly a testament to Jessica's amazing spirit. She was and is so loved by everyone.

She has touched so many lives through her teaching, giving, and coaching—and then, through this journey. I am honored to call her daughter. She's God's daughter too. I knew that He loved her and was with her and us every step of the way. So many people have asked me why this would happen to such a great person and family. I don't have that answer—yet.

Later that day, Jess was weaned off much of her sedation. This morning, her dad and I were holding her hands and talking to her. When I let go of her hand, she lifted her arm purposefully as if she were trying to find my hand. She also moved her head. This was great news! However, she still had to rest very quietly. They didn't want too much stimulation yet.

What I knew in my heart is that this was Jess's way of telling us she's here, and she's fighting. On the way into the hospital, I saw a sign that said, "Happy people are often thankful, but thankful people are always happy." I was thankful for the little gestures of a moving hand and a turning head. I was grateful that Jess was fighting a good fight. I don't know if happiness had crept in yet, but hope had.

Day 7

November 2, 2015

Day 7 was the hardest so far. I didn't really know why. I just knew that I was not able to look at all the pictures of my beautiful daughter with her baby girl without bursting into tears. My heart was broken into a million pieces. I yelled at the guy in the hospital, taking my information this morning because he didn't smile or say, "Have a nice day." I wanted to shake him and tell him to smile at everyone because you don't know what each person walking through that door is dealing with. God, we take so much for granted. I was thankful today that my daughter blinked when the nurse told her I was there. She blinked! Does anyone get this? I was thankful for a blink.

So, all of you reading this get down on your knees tonight and thank God if your child was able to smile at you today. Thank Him if you heard your child's voice. Thank Him if you felt your child's touch. I was not able to thank Him for those things that night. The sadness was like a great big wave threatening to crash into me and crush me, but I wouldn't let it.

Maybe I couldn't thank him for Jessica's smile, touch, or voice, but I could thank Him for the strength I knew He was giving all of us to see Jessica through this. I could thank Him for the countless blessings that

Jessica's journey has brought to this community. I could thank him for all the people that were walking with us— all of you reading this story. Jess was fighting hard. I knew she was there and wanted so much to come back to us. That evening, there was a gathering to pray for Jessica at 6:30 at the hospital. I asked everyone to bring a candle so we could show the world her shining light.

Day 9

More Bunches of Sunshine

November 4, 2015

I'm not going to lie and say that my faith remained unshaken through all of this. What I can say is that Jess's faith and the faith of the friends and family surrounding her were enormous. Being surrounded by people of faith was a help to our family.

My beautiful granddaughter, Eva, always brings me pictures when she comes to my house, and she tells me that they are full of "bunches of sunshine." Today, I told Jessica that Eva is sending her bunches of sunshine, and she immediately responded with a blink. I'm going to take that as a sign that God's got this. Eva has been so strong and brave, like her mommy. She knows Mommy's in the hospital getting fixed.

Today, Jessica is resting. She is on less sedation and is continuing with pain medicine. The drain has been removed from her head. She has had no seizure activity and no further strokes. I watched her fight the nurse yesterday when Jess was trying to pull the breathing tube out, and the nurse was trying to stop her. The nurse commented on how strong Jessica is.

We all know how strong Jessica is! When my faith is shaken, I just keep thinking about my beautiful Eva, and

I look for bunches of sunshine wherever I can. Today, I found bunches of sunshine in a blink. Maybe tomorrow it will be in a touch. Someday I'll find bunches of sunshine in Jessica's voice.

Chapter 3

UNtruths

The Farm

December 2016

I often think about Eva and how much she must have been wondering what happened to her mommy. When this happened to Jess, I wanted so much to be with Eva and explain to her that her mommy was very sick. I wanted to tell her the truth. I wanted her to know that she was surrounded by people who loved her and would take care of her no matter what. Mostly, I just wanted to hold her close and sing her favorite lullaby and pray with her that Mommy would come back to her.

Unfortunately, I was not able to be near Eva. I might as well have been on the other side of the world because Aaron was not going to let Eva be exposed to anyone who might speak the truth to her. He was going to protect her at all costs. I wasn't very far away from Eva at the hospital, and I could have pushed the issue.

In fact, I tried to push the issue. I tried to involve the child life specialists, but Aaron would have none of it. I was with Jess day and night and didn't get to see Eva for weeks on end. After about three weeks at the first hospital, I went with Jess to the second hospital that was six hours away. I never even spoke to Eva on the phone during those days. No one in our family had any access to Eva. Aaron and his mother were caring for Eva—period.

Although I wrote in my CaringBridge post that Aaron was doing a great job with Eva, I had personal concerns that I did not wish to disclose publicly. I knew Aaron was not truthful with Eva when he told her that Mommy had a boo-boo. I felt Eva's pain and her fear as if it were my own like I had been tossed into some weird time-warp machine that took me back to my childhood. I tried to explain to Aaron the importance of truthfulness with Eva.

I understood that Aaron did not want Eva to see her mommy with IV tubes and a machine breathing for her. I realized how scary that would be, but I didn't understand his reluctance to involve the child-life specialists at the hospital or his unwillingness to bring Eva with him to the prayer vigil for her mommy that was held outside the hospital.

Many months later, after Jess was no longer hooked up to the ventilator and other machines, Jack and I begged Aaron to bring Eva to see her mommy, but he never relented. There were many things about Jess that Eva would have to learn to accept. Jack and I both felt it was vitally important that Eva understand the changes in her mommy. She needed to know that the mommy who left to go on a run one day was not going to be the same mommy that would be coming home to her.

The mommy that was coming home to Eva would not be able to walk, let alone run. Eva was used to having Jessica take her to the park, but Jess couldn't drive any longer. Jess had to wear a helmet now to protect her head. Jess couldn't use her left arm, hand, or leg. Jess couldn't communicate like she used to, and she had memory problems. I believe these were things that Eva needed to know now. Jack and I felt that they needed to be addressed by a professional counselor so Eva could process everything before Jessica came home.

Aaron never yielded. He and I frequently butted heads over the way to handle Jess's illness with Eva. By the time Jess was moved to Holy Cross Rehabilitation Hospital, we had already had our share of arguments. The arguments were never in front of Jess. We often argued in the ICU waiting room, hospital hallways, or the hospital parking lot. It seemed whenever we were out of earshot of Jess, we'd resume the argument right where we left off.

It was as if the only way we communicated with each other was through verbal lashings. I don't know if it was the stress of the entire situation. Whatever the reason, I think people were secretly placing bets on who would win the current showdown. I guess it depended on who was keeping score, but no matter what the score, in my mind, there were always two clear losers: Jess and Eva.

Our incessant fights at Holy Cross Hospital became legendary. We even got kicked out of Jessica's room once while she was out at therapy. That episode is the one that has stuck in my head. I even remember most of the words that we exchanged. It's as if this one event sums up much of our relationship during Jess's illness, both at the first hospital and then at Holy Cross Hospital.

Reflection

Jack, on the other hand, was far more subtle than I when it came to expressing our concerns about Eva. Jack would ask Aaron direct questions such as, "What is the name of the child psychologist you spoke with?" Aaron would answer that he has a friend who is a child psychologist, ducking and dodging Jack's questions. Jack, the quiet calm assessor, was like a boxer sizing up the situation and waiting for the right time to strike. I was not so patient!

Dr. Wishywashy

I remember the scene well. Aaron was standing by the window on the far side of the room when I returned from taking Jess to therapy. I blocked the door as he turned to me with a look of disdain as if he already knew I was going to bring up Eva. I did.

"Are you at least going to allow the two of them to FaceTime?" I asked.

"Why?" he retorted, "Jess won't remember it anyway, and it will just upset Eva."

"What the hell is wrong with you?" I snapped. "Eva needs her mommy."

"You don't know what you're talking about!" he shouted. "I've consulted a child psychologist, and he says that I should not allow her to see Jess like this."

"Like what?" I yelled. "Like the mother that she is going to have from now on? This is who Jess is, Aaron. She will get better, but it will be a slow progression. You need to let Eva see her mommy just as she is. Please, just let them FaceTime. Jess cries for Eva every morning and every night before going to sleep. She tells me that she had nightmares about never seeing Eva again. This is awful, Aaron. It's awful for Jess, and it's awful for Eva!"

"Eva is perfectly happy!" Aaron shouted back at me. "Why would I put her through this? Besides, Jess may very well be walking by the time she leaves here."

"You're delusional!" I cried. "You are not here every day watching Jess struggle. She's not walking out of here, Aaron. It's time you face that. It's time you face the fact that your family will be different now. Face the fact that your daughter needs her mommy, and Jess needs to see Eva."

Our voices were getting louder and louder. The argument was spilling into the hallway, and I wasn't allowing Aaron an escape route. Suddenly I heard someone behind me.

"One of you will have to leave now!" The no-nonsense nurse stood in the doorway with her arms folded across her chest. Aaron quickly discerned this was his opportunity to leave. He scrambled sideways between the nurse and me, avoiding eye contact with either of us.

Aaron was out the door and in the elevator in less than ten seconds. After his departure, there was a loud crashing noise that came from the elevator. I'm not sure, but I would venture a guess that the cracks in the elevator mirror and slivers of glass gleaming on the elevator floor had something to do with Aaron's disappearing act and the loud crash we all heard that morning.

Aaron was gone for hours after our heated exchange. When he returned, he acted as if nothing had ever happened between us. In his mind, the score was settled. Aaron added another "W" to his win column. I just felt drained and sad for both Jessica and Eva (and I might have had a little sadness leftover for Aaron).

I may have lost this battle, but Aaron didn't know me well if he thought that I was giving up the fight. He never brought Eva to the hospital, and I never stopped fighting for her and Jess to see each other.

Jess's average day at Holy Cross Hospital was filled with therapy sessions: Occupational Therapy, Physical Therapy, Cognitive Therapy, Recreational Therapy, Speech Therapy—every kind of therapy imaginable. Working alongside Jess's team of therapists was a team of medical doctors and one psychologist. The medical doctors evaluated Jess once a week, sometimes more frequently.

The psychologist never met with Jess, despite the frequent assertions of concern from the nursing staff and me over Jess's anxiety about not seeing her daughter. Jess woke up every morning crying for Eva and went to bed every night praying she'd see her daughter soon. Despite Jess's frequent emotional breakdowns, the psychologist did not see the necessity to speak with Jess or me.

The staff became so concerned about Jess that they asked the psychologist to evaluate her for depression. I was present for the evaluation, which consisted of a five-minute conversation between Jess and the psychologist. The psychologist asked her how she was doing and if she had any concerns. Jess, who was unable to express her feelings verbally at this point in her recovery, answered with two words: "fine" and "no."

I couldn't believe this "evaluation," and I asked the psychologist to speak with me for a moment in the hallway. The conversation that followed went something like this:

Me: You didn't ask Jess about Eva.

Dr.: I didn't want to upset her.

Me: How can you evaluate her state of mind in five minutes and not bring up the one thing that is making her so depressed?

Dr.: I have the reports from the staff, and I can make a determination based on their observations. Jess isn't really at a point where she can express her emotions yet.

Me: So, all the times she cries for her daughter does not count as expressing her emotions?

Dr.: I will put her on an antidepressant.

Me: The only antidepressant that will work for Jess would be telling her husband that it's high time he allowed Eva and Jess to see each other.

Dr.: This is ultimately Aaron's decision, and we have to abide by his wishes.

Me: Why?

Dr.: Why don't we schedule a meeting between you and Aaron, and we can discuss this in my office?

Me: What about Jess? Won't she be at the meeting?

Dr.: She's not able to communicate well enough yet.

Me: Okay, so you evaluated that she is not able to communicate well enough yet in exactly five minutes of meeting with Jess?

Dr.: I will try to meet with her again before I meet with you and Aaron.

Me: Great. I'm certain that Jess will feel like opening up to you since you've spent so much time with her!

I gave the resident psychologist a nickname after our little discussion in the hallway—Dr. Wishywashy because she refused to stand up for Jessica. Not long after her "evaluation" of Jess, Dr. Wishywashy called Aaron and me into her office. She didn't find the time to meet Jess again, so she relied on her notes from the nursing staff to begin the meeting.

"The nurses and CNAs have stated that Jess wakes up every morning asking for Eva," Dr. Wishywashy reported.

"Not 'asking,' crying!" I countered. "She also goes to sleep crying for Eva every night."

"I don't think Eva needs to see her mother like this," Aaron said.

"Like what?" I could feel the heat rising in my cheeks, making them as red-hot as my anger.

After the heated exchange became a wildfire and almost burned down the office of Dr. Wishywashy, she called a truce. Dr. Wishywashy soothed and coaxed until Aaron finally acquiesced and agreed to allow Jessica and Eva to FaceTime. I wanted to pull out my scorecard and add a "W" to my column, but I still didn't feel like this was a win. It was a tiny victory, but I'd take it. I wished Jess had been present in Dr. Wishywashy's office to witness this, but Jess's opinion didn't matter to Dr. Wishywashy or Aaron.

When I returned to Jess's room, I told her the news that she would be able to see Eva on a FaceTime call. It's the first time I saw her eyes light up before they welled with tears.

"When?" she asked as the tears rolled down her face and spilled off her nose.

"I hope it will be soon," I answered. "Aaron has a long drive home. I don't know if he'll have her call tonight or sometime later this week."

I couldn't give Jess any more information since I didn't know Aaron's timeline. I assumed he would come into her room and give her the news himself. Unfortunately, Jess didn't comprehend time at this point. To Jess, a day could last an hour or a week. Her cognitive development still had a long way to go, but she had come so far since the day we arrived.

I had to hold tight to that knowledge—she's come so far! Now, she'd have to wait for Aaron to cave and allow the phone call to happen. I had to hope that he understood how much this meant to Jess and would have Eva call as soon as possible. I wanted to believe in him. Knowing that he held all the power to determine when this FaceTime call would transpire made me crazy, but I had to focus on Jess and not my anger at him.

The only hope Aaron gave Jess was to tell her that he was going to have Eva FaceTime soon. That was it. Soon. Jess no more understood "soon" as she understood "in an hour" or "tomorrow." "After dinner" was much more concrete and understandable for her. So, I told Jess that Eva would call after Jess had dinner. I didn't know what else to say to her. It was three days of "after dinner" before the call came. Three days of waiting. Three days of crying. Three days of agony, but eventually, the magic of FaceTime transported the enchantment of Eva through the phone.

I cannot express the joy that filled Jess when I told her the "Eva call" was finally happening! It was so touching and more than a little heartbreaking to see the expression on Jess's face. At first, her face lit up. Then, she got a faraway look in her eyes, and I knew she wished that she could hold her baby girl in her arms. Yet, Jess was so happy to see Eva, even if it was just through the phone. It lifted her spirits so much. I sat off to the side sobbing as I listened to the two of them discussing such riveting topics as what they had for dinner.

Of course, Eva handled everything in stride. It was clear that she was very excited to talk to her mommy finally. I didn't sense any great anxiety on Eva's part. I'd say she was more curious than anything.

"Where are you?"

Unfortunately, Jess was unable to say exactly where she was because her cognitive development hadn't reached a point where she understood place and time. I wiped my snotty nose and jumped into the picture to fill in some of the blanks.

"Nana!" Eva looked so surprised to see me.

It hadn't occurred to me that Eva wouldn't know that Nana was with Mommy.

"Hello, beautiful," I said in a cheerful voice. "I'm at the hospital with Mommy."

"Why are you crying?" asked Eva.

"These are my happy tears," I explained. "I'm so happy that you are talking to Mommy."

"Me too," said Eva.

"Here's Mommy," I said as I handed the phone back to Jess. "I love you, Eva."

Jess couldn't stop smiling as she took the phone back. Her joy was contagious, and Eva started laughing.

"Why are you wearing a helmet, Mommy?" she asked.

Jess explained that the helmet was protecting her brain and that she wouldn't have to wear it forever. Eva decided that she wanted a helmet too, and they would decorate their helmets in pink flowers when Mommy came home. In true three-year-old fashion, the conversation lasted about two minutes before Eva's attention was drawn to her dolls and her imaginary friends. They were waiting for their "teacher" (Eva) to return to class. Jess handled the call with a marvelous grace. After she hung up, she cried. I cried with her.

Jess got a phone call from Eva every day after that. The Eva calls helped Jess get through her therapy sessions because she knew the better she got, the quicker she'd be going home to Eva.

Reflection

I think I had more difficulty than Jess processing the Eva calls because I knew how hard life was going to be for the two of them when Jess returned home. I was hopeful that Aaron would be able to handle the new relationships they would all have to develop; still, I didn't know how he would do it alone. In so many ways, this situation reminded me of my childhood and my father's inability to explain the loss to his children. Eva, in many ways, lost the mother she knew, and Aaron would have to address this reality with her. I feared for all of them because I didn't think Aaron was able to comprehend the gravity of their circumstances.

Chapter 4

UNforgiving

The Farm

December 2016

The anger inside me even a year after Jess's brain aneurysm still boiled over and mixed with deep sadness that was as raw as a visceral smell. An awful smell, a rotting smell. My soul was rotting, and I didn't know how to stop it.

I wish I could say that God had blessed me with wisdom beyond my years. I wish I could say that he had blessed me with wisdom that calms my soul with healing words. I wish I could say that the wise words are as plentiful as the age spots on my grandma hands. If only, I had a wise word for every age spot. Oh well. I don't.

I'm not like my grandma, who imparted wisdom as she taught me the art of making fancy drip castles by dripping wet sand off my thumb. Grandma taught me so much about life during those summer days I spent with her in Atlantic City. I learned how to appreciate the beauty of the crashing waves on the sand. I learned to appreciate the hours of silence between us occasionally broken by the squawk of a gull. I absorbed it all even when I didn't know I was doing it.

The last time I saw Grandma, she told me something very wise as we sat on the beach looking out into the vast Atlantic. I knew what she was saying was profound and that I should remember it, but I didn't. Somehow, I sensed that this might be my last time with her. I felt like we were saying goodbye, but I didn't know why I felt that way. She wasn't sick. She wasn't sickly—she was full of life and happier than I ever remember her being.

I remember getting on the bus to go home and looking out at her waving goodbye and thinking, *I'm going to miss her so much!* During the three-hour bus ride home, I kept reminding myself, *I must never forget what she told me today.* I wish now that I could remember what she said to me.

Three weeks later, I was visiting my aunt when she got a phone call. I knew that the phone call was not good news by the look on my aunt's face. Before she hung up, I felt in my gut that the call was about my grandma. To this day, I cannot explain how or why I knew these things—premonitions, I guess.

The call was from the building manager at my grandmother's apartment. She had been making chicken soup, something she always did when one of us was feeling under the weather. The pan caught on fire on her stove, and the fire alarm alerted the building manager. He found her sitting on the couch in her apartment. He said that he didn't even realize she was dead at first. The autopsy said she died of a heart attack. She was seventy-two years old and had never been sick a day in her life.

Now, I'm a grandma, and I still search for wisdom. I want to take my granddaughter in my arms and fill her with the same kind of great insights my grandmother poured into me, but she'd probably forget it anyway. What's that saying? Youth is wasted on the young. When we're young, we don't realize how much time we spend on foolish follies. When we're old, we don't realize that the young'uns aren't listening to us anyway, and they have to make their own mistakes.

They may hear a few words here and there. They might even learn a lesson once in a while. However, they do watch us. They watch everything. That's why I think it is more important to be attentive to our actions as adults and not our words. That's my wisdom for the day.

I wish I could say that my actions and my words towards my son-in-law were wise. They weren't.

Since I'm thinking about sitting with my grandma building sandcastles at the beach, I'll use a beach analogy for Aaron. He and I swam in the shallows most of the time. Still waters run deep, or so I'm told. Shallow waters are just that—shallow. Aaron didn't share his feelings much except to express how much pain my daughter caused him with this horrible illness. "I can't believe this has happened to me!" was his favorite rant. I ignored him mostly except when confronted with the obvious elephant in the room, Jessica crying because she missed Eva so much.

The eruption in the shallows was not usually caused by a man-eating shark, although that's not a bad idea. No, the eruption was usually caused by me yelling obscenities at Aaron for not seeing the obvious distress he was causing Jessica. Of course, I always timed my explosions when Jessica was out of her room at therapy, and Aaron was usually packing to leave. I knew he'd be gone soon on his five-hour journey home, and I wanted him to be thinking long and hard about the pain he was causing his wife.

There was a part of me that thought Aaron didn't think long and hard about anything not having to do directly with Aaron. His wife was an afterthought. I don't know that he ever thought about Eva missing her mom. I don't think Aaron possessed that kind of empathy.

Frankly, I don't think Aaron had any compassion for anyone. He certainly didn't respect me, and I don't believe that he was capable of loving Jess after her aneurysm. I want to add: But that's neither here nor there, but that's not true. His lack of empathy is here and there and everywhere!

Indeed, Aaron's inability to empathize is an essential theme throughout this story. Maybe I've been looking at him all wrong. Perhaps I could not see him as a person who just couldn't handle what was happening to his wife and his neat little life. I'm not a psychologist, but I've psychoanalyzed Aaron. Perhaps if I understood him better, I'd approach him differently. My attempts to appeal to Aaron's sense of decency and pleading for him to see what he is doing to Jessica and Eva are futile. Like trying to put a square peg in a round hole. So, what do I do? Maybe nothing.

Aaron, thankfully, is out of Jessica's life now except for the sad reality that he is Eva's father. I can't think about Aaron anymore, or I'll be consumed with thoughts of a man-eating shark in the shallows devouring him, piece by piece. Small bites, please—not one big gulp.

Reflection

I gulp. Why? Why do I entertain such vile thoughts? They'll just hurt me in the long run.

I'll think about Eva for a few minutes. Thoughts of Eva always make me smile. I took care of her when she was an infant until she was about two. I have great memories of Eva and me and all the fun things we did together. Whenever we went swimming, she would say, "I need my bathing soup and sun scream." Sometimes, looking back on those happy memories with Eva gives me just the boost I need.

Chapter 5

UNrelenting

Bathing Soup and Sun Scream

Something magical happens when you're a grandma. I'm called Nana. To some, Nana conjures up images of an old lady sitting in a rocking chair reading books and singing to a content toddler in her lap. Not this Nana! This Nana is very busy indeed. There are a few times when a good book and a comfy rocking chair serve their purpose for a few seconds. But when two-year-old Eva is in the house, we're more likely to be rocking and rolling than rocking and dozing.

Magically, Nana's knee finds a way to keep up the pace (even though I've had a knee replacement). My energy level gets a boost out of nowhere, and I can Nay Nay and Whip my way into a frenzy dancing to Janis Joplin on the old record player. There is no slide too tall nor fort too low for Nana. The super-human strength even holds up when Eva suddenly has to ride on Nana's shoulders during the longest hike ever into the pasture to find the elusive crowing rooster.

What is it about being a nana that brings out this magical vigor? I think it is a mixture of bathing soup and sun scream. Every time Eva and I are together, we laugh. We laugh our way through Miss Eva's Whip and Nay Nay dance lessons. We laugh as we sail over rough seas in the S. S. Sofa. We laugh at bubble bath beards and edible cow pies (Eva's favorite imaginary snack). There is nothing too crazy for Nana and Eva: between finding the hippopotamus hiding in the closet to dragging the giraffe out from under the bed, we laugh our way through the day.

I think about spending summers at the Jersey Shore in Atlantic City with my grandma. We'd spend hours on the beach making our elaborate drip castles, just grandma and me. It seemed that time stood still during those hours that we let the sand drip off our fingers, creating beautiful palaces for imaginary princes and princesses. Sometimes we talked, sometimes we just dripped our castle—no words necessary.

There are days I wish that I could gather up those grains of sand and turn them into seconds. If I did, I bet I would have enough seconds to fill up another lifetime with my grandma. She didn't watch the clock worrying that we were frittering away our time. Even though she had arthritic fingers, she never once told me that we needed to stop building drip castles. She knew the secret of grandma strength—laugh, dream, imagine, and love.

Today, I was getting Eva ready for a day at the beach with Nana. As we were gathering up our pails and shovels for our drip castles, Eva reminded me that she needed to get her bathing soup on and that I need to pack the sun scream. I laughed.

Chapter 6

UNhopeful

The Farm

December 2016

That smell is back. Pigs. Pigs, horses, horse manure, and dog. All the smells of the farm. Why can't I smell Juicy Fruit gum? That smell bypasses all the pathways in my brain and goes directly to the longing emotion. I don't long to chew Juicy Fruit gum. I long for its smell. That smell was one of the things that made me smile when I was three. I remember it so well. I remember the spot of sunlight, much like the spot in front of me now. It shone on the floor in front of the desk where the Juicy Fruit gum was kept.

I always sat in the spot of sunlight when I opened the third drawer. I was just able to reach the drawer and pull it open enough to release the smell. That's it. I'd sit on the sun-spotted floor and smell Juicy Fruit gum until my aunt appeared and swept me up into her arms to start the day. I don't know why that memory has stuck to my soul even after all these years. Perhaps my soul longs for the simplicity of the Juicy Fruit gum smell. It matches the simplicity of the sunlit moment with no worries, and no one telling me that Mommy went to the store.

I move from my perch and sit on the leaf-covered sunspot now. Hope fills me, hoping for the smell of Juicy Fruit gum. I'm hoping for my aunt to scoop me up and hold me. I'm hoping for my grandma's wise words to come upon me. I'm hoping for God to show up. All around me, I see nature. I don't see streets or cars. I don't hear people yelling. I don't hear anything manmade. All I hear are God noises. All I see are God's creations, yet I still wait for Him to show up.

Maybe He's already here, says the small voice that I want to ignore. That would be too simple. God can't just be here. If He were here, big things would be happening! God doesn't make small, quiet entrances. He burns bushes and sends angels. He tells us truths in the Bible. I don't even have my Bible out here.

I move from the sunlight—enough of this ruminating. Hope isn't going to find me today. Anyway, I want to be hopeless right now. I want to wallow in self-pity. Can't I wallow for a while? I should join the pigs. The pigs are champion wallowers.

I walk away from the light and find another branch. I think about wallowing. I'm not happy—I should be happy. I have all this land, five acres, to be exact. That doesn't seem like a lot until you have to mow it and care for it. Then there's the barn and the house and all the animals that come with it: five acres, two donkeys, four chickens, one horse, two dogs, and a cat. I'm not the only one taking care of this place. It's Jack and I. We also have a few kids—grown mostly.

Chapter 7

UNbelievable

Jessica's Homecoming

One child came back, though. She didn't come back on her own. She was dropped off. She was left here—discarded like clothes left at Goodwill. There was no goodwill here when Jessica was discarded. We didn't thank Aaron for his donation. It was more like we kicked him to the curb, or should I say our daughter Emily kicked him to the curb.

Before Emily disposed of him, Aaron and his Aunt Cathy also brought Eva to our house to spend the weekend with Jess and us. Jess was already here because I had insisted on picking her up the day before from Aaron's mother's house.

We were done playing games with Aaron because he was doing the same thing to us as he had done to Eva. He was isolating us from our daughter and not allowing us access to her at his mother's house, where she returned after her release from the hospital. We were very close to calling the authorities to investigate possible neglect of our daughter.

It was an uphill battle for us to see Jess, and Aaron always claimed Jess's phone was not working, so we couldn't even call her. We emailed him and texted him daily, and he often ignored us. When he did email us, he frequently mentioned putting Jess in a skilled nursing facility.

Knowing that we were very concerned about our daughter's wellbeing, Aaron finally relented and agreed to a meeting at our house on September 24, 2016. I'm sure Aaron felt like he was walking into the lion's den (so to speak) since he clearly viewed us as his enemies.

When we had the meeting, it was just one month shy of a year after Jess's brain aneurysm, yet it felt more like ten years. Aaron sat at our large dining room table with his disabled wife sitting directly across from him in her wheelchair. It was a heart-wrenching picture. Jess looked at Aaron with hope-filled eyes. I don't believe she had any idea what was coming. There was an innocence about Jess since the aneurysm, and she gave everyone the impression that she was very content with her life.

Jess was always happy even as a child. Now that she is getting better, it's as if her happiness has more meaning—joy. Joy is what Jess is filled with. I guess it is the kind of joy that comes from knowing life is so precious that every minute must be savored. She looked joyful as well as hopeful. I couldn't help but think that Aaron would be moved by Jess's upbeat mood as she sat across from him. I don't know why I thought that!

Looking back now, I think part of Jess's joy came from getting out of her mother-in-law's house and coming to our home. I'm sure that she was thrilled to have Eva with her too. Honestly, I think she was relieved and excited about the prospect of being in our home with her daughter for the entire weekend.

Aaron, on the other hand, looked dark and brooding. I didn't see any warmth or compassion in Aaron's eyes. Of course, I knew I wouldn't see any sympathy because I didn't believe he could feel compassion. Believing he lacked empathy and seeing it in action are two different things, though. It's hard to describe black eyes that show no emotion. It's like looking into a stagnant puddle of black road runoff.

Jack and I were flanking Aaron on either side. At this point, we had no idea that Aaron was going to mention the "D" word. We just wanted to know what his reasoning was for keeping our daughter from us. We were willing to offer three days a week of care for Jess in lieu of a skilled nursing facility. We wanted Jessica to be a part of the conversation because she was perfectly capable of understanding Aaron's plan for her life.

Our main goal was for Jessica to know that we very much wanted to be a part of her life. We would do whatever it took to see to it that she was surrounded by people who love her—not nurses, skilled though they may be.

We thought Aaron might ask us to keep Jess at our home overnight so he could have respite time. We were prepared to offer whatever assistance necessary. We were not prepared for the bomb Aaron was about to drop.

Aaron's Aunt Cathy perched at the far end of the table. She reminded me of an ostrich with her long neck, beady eyes, beak-like nose, and close-cropped feathery reddish hair. Cathy's expression was dispassionate but not uninterested. Initially, I wondered why she accompanied Aaron, but I soon realized that she was part of the plan, and this "meeting" was as rehearsed as a Broadway play—right down to Aaron's fake sobbing in his hands (something we had already witnessed first-hand at the hospital).

Jack and I began the discussion by asking Aaron to explain to us why we hadn't been able to see Jess regularly since she'd been living at his mom's house. He began his feeble reply when Jess cut him off by saying she didn't know he was keeping us from her. As the discussion progressed, we asked Aaron to explain why Jess wasn't getting Botox treatments for her hand and foot. He had plenty of fundraiser money to pay for the treatment, even if it wasn't completely covered by insurance. When the conversation turned to Jess's disability checks that she'd been receiving since April, the aunt motioned Jack outside.

Outside, "Ostrich Aunt" proceeded to tell Jack that the disability money, $1,600.00/month, went to Jess's living expenses. Her pre-rehearsed dialogue included the fact that Aaron was very concerned because all Jess and Aaron's church friends had deserted them. Cathy confided that Jess's women friends could not handle the disability and felt uncomfortable around Jess. I'm sure Jack was very moved by her revelations.

After Jack and Aunty went outside, Aaron placed his head in his hands and began to fake cry. I rolled my eyes. I wasn't buying any of it. Jess sat in her wheelchair, dumbfounded by what Aaron said through his "sobs."

My jaw dropped as I listened to Aaron.

"I have to divorce you; don't you see? It's the best thing for you. I make too much money, but if I divorce you, then you can get Medicaid and Medicare. They'll pay for you to go to a skilled nursing facility where you can get round-the-clock care. I'll bring Eva to visit you every day."

Before the meeting, we helped Jess compose a list of questions for Aaron. Her list was sitting on the hutch by the table. I handed Jess the list and listened to their exchange. I couldn't believe what I was seeing and hearing! Jess, through her real tears, was reading her list of questions, and Aaron was matter-of-factly answering as if Jess was asking him about the weather. I was becoming more and more furious with Aaron as he spoke. Looking at Jess, my fury quickly turned to heartbreak.

It was so painful as a mother to see and hear this scene playing out at my dining room table. There was something so wrong about this! I didn't speak—I couldn't. Their voices droned on in my head, sounding more and more like two people speaking underwater.

Jess: Why do you want to put me in a nursing home?

Aaron: Not a nursing home, a skilled nursing facility where you will get round-the-clock care. A facility where you will not be watching HGTV for 13 hours a day. I'll bring Eva to visit.

Jess: Will you go to counseling?

Aaron: Why? What is our marriage anyway? I'm just your caregiver.

Jess: What are your plans for Eva?

Aaron: She'll live with me, and we'll come to visit you.

Jess: What are your plans for the future of our family?

Aaron: I'll divorce you because then you will qualify for Medicare and Medicaid and will be able to go into the skilled nursing facility to get the help you need. I've looked into lots of facilities. I have a list in a notebook on my desk at work....

Just as I was about to slap Aaron, Emily and Eva came into the house. Emily quickly sized up the situation. She took one look at her sister, and I knew that the slap I was about to administer would more than likely come from Emily.

Emily is a feisty one. She's short on words and short in stature, but she has a presence about her.

"I think you're done here, Aaron!" she shouted at the pretend-sobbing figure sitting across from his real-sobbing wife. "Get out!"

Aaron quickly stood. He took his leave without even so much as a glance back at his devastated wife. Aaron didn't have any parting words, but Jack did. As Aaron emerged from the house, he practically ran into Ostrich Aunt and Jack still talking on the porch. Emily followed Aaron like a little yappy dog nipping at his heels. Jack sized up the situation and yelled at Aaron's departing figure, "You're quite the Christian guy, Aaron!"

Aaron turned, puffed up his chest gorilla-like, and tried to look menacing. The look he was going for didn't stick. Jack's look withered Aaron immediately, and I guess Aaron thought better of taking on an angry ex-wrestler father. Instead, he escaped to his car with Ostrich Aunt on his heels.

Thankfully, it had been pre-arranged that Eva was spending the weekend with us, and Emily's hard look told Aaron that Eva would not be leaving with him. The whole scene was infuriating and heartbreaking, but I was thankful that Jess and Eva were with us. I knew that Jess would now be our full-time charge. There was no way she'd return to the soon to be ex-mother-in-law and no way she'd be going into a skilled nursing facility.

I wasn't sure what was going to happen with Eva, but I knew that we'd fight Aaron tooth and nail for Jess to get shared custody. If he thought he was just going to walk away from his wife, he had another thing coming!

We watched Aaron and Ostrich Aunt make their escape. Then, Emily grabbed Eva's hand, and they went inside to play school.

Chapter 8

UNstoppable

Emily

Emily has always been a tough cookie. She's not one to give up on anything. I remember when years ago, Emily got a new car that had a manual transmission. This, of course, meant that we had to teach her how to shift. Easy, right? Wrong. I don't remember my dad teaching me how to shift gears, but I know I had to be easier to teach than Emily!

Back in my day, we all learned how to drive stick shifts. I guess it was mandatory since most of the cars we owned still had manual transmissions. I remember one time I had to drive a dump truck. It was full of horse manure from the farm where I worked. I was tasked with taking the truck down the highway to the mushroom farm. I thought I was shifting the gear when I inadvertently pulled back on the lever for the dumping mechanism. There I was driving down the road, oblivious to the fact that I was dumping a load of horse manure in my wake!

Now, twenty years later, I was with my 17-year-old daughter trying to teach her how to shift. At least, it wasn't a dump truck full of poop. I told Emily the story of the dump truck as we made our way to her new car. She didn't appear to be amused. She looked a little scared as she took her place in the driver's seat. I just knew as I buckled my seat belt that I'd have to write a story about teaching Emily to shift.

Shift

The word shift has so many meanings in life. You can shift your opinion about something, shift your lifestyle, shift your attitude, and shift from one stage of life to another. Constant shifting is a balancing act. I experienced a shift of my own when I threw the car keys over to my 17-year-old daughter. As I threw her the keys, I realized that my little girl had suddenly grown up. Our roles as mother and daughter had made a profound and lasting shift. It was as if the baton were passed in the race of life.

As the keys flew through the air, I felt as though I had been thrown into some weird time-warp where my child transformed from little girl to teenager to young woman. The seventeen years of life we'd spent together seemed to flash before me in the sunlight reflecting on the silver.

As I took my place in the car next to her, I wondered when she grew up. When did my little girl who toddled around the house grow into this beautiful young woman getting behind the wheel? Wasn't it just yesterday that I was rocking her and singing, "Puff the Magic Dragon"? Was it that long ago that I pushed her on a swing and caught her at the bottom of a slide?

I remember as if it were yesterday, her curls bobbing up and down as she rode her rocking horse to some imagined destination. It wasn't long after that she was riding a real horse with me leading her through the pasture. Then, one day, she took the reins all by herself.

My brain was screaming: Too soon—she cannot grow up yet! I don't know if I've taught her everything she needs to know. She's still just a baby, isn't she? No. No, today is the day that everything shifts. Today, we are making our maiden stick shift voyage on the road (after many weeks of lurching through our pasture). It is another cruel reminder that my little Emily is becoming a grown woman. Goodness knows, she could have children of her own soon, and I could be a grandma. Grandma! I'm too young for that.

I was quickly brought back to reality when I heard the grinding of first gear, and I barely escaped whiplash as we jerked down the road.

"Emily," I said calmly, "ease your foot off the clutch."

"I am, Mom," came her exasperated reply. I could see the tears begin to well in her eyes. "I've got it, Mom!"

"Okay, honey," I said through clenched teeth, "let's just get to Walmart and back."

Walmart was about two miles down the road. We hit three stoplights along the way. There are many things that I am thankful for in my life, but on this day, I was grateful that we have very flat roads. We only stalled about four times, and my life only flashed before my eyes one time when we were turning into Walmart, and the oncoming traffic was fast approaching our stalled car.

Emily's parking of the car presented its set of challenges. We found a spot fairly far away with only one car to the right of the parking space. Emily slowly began to ease her foot off the clutch in first gear, and we lurched and stalled, lurched and stalled until, finally, the car was far enough in the parking space that I deemed it parked. We got out of the vehicle. Emily went first, and I followed behind her (getting out on her side because I couldn't open my door).

We inspected the parking job, and I told her how proud I was of her, even if the car was a bit crooked. She gave me an exasperated look reserved for me. It's the modified eye roll that says, Mom, I know you're lying just to make me feel better.

Isn't that what moms are supposed to do? Isn't my job to build up her confidence so that one day she'll get into the stick shift car and venture out on her own while I sit home, waiting anxiously by the phone for her call telling me she's arrived safely?

As we browsed through Walmart, I worried about our return trip: Would she be able to back out of the parking space? Would she stall in the middle of the intersection, leaving the busy store?

Worry, worry, worry!

It reminded me of her sixteenth birthday when I naively took her and a "few" of her friends to the beach and rented a room for the night. I had no idea what I was getting myself into. The six friends grew to about sixteen friends (including boys), and I was entrusted with keeping all the girls safe. Needless to say, it was not the smartest thing I have ever done. Emily still reminds me of my overbearing presence.

The icing on the cake was when she called me from the hospital after I let her stay with her older sister to go out on a jet ski. She had fallen off the back of the jet ski, hit her chin on the way down, and was in the process of getting her chin stitched up.

Sometimes, when I look back over the years, I wonder how I survived motherhood and all its challenges. I wonder about all the times I flew by the seat of my pants, second-guessing my decisions. *Did I give them all enough guidance? Did I give them too much guidance? Did I allow them the freedom to make mistakes? Did I prepare them for all the shifts they will face in their lives?*

We made our way back to the car. Emily looked at me as we settled in and said, "I got this, Mom."

"I know you do," I said as my eyes misted. "I know you will do just fine."

I glanced over at her and, just for a moment, I thought I saw that curly-top toddler. I blinked, and I saw the little girl on top of her pony. One more blink, and I saw her running down the soccer field. *Where did the time go?* I wondered. Then, I was brought back to reality as the car lurched backward out of the parking space.

"Ease that foot off the clutch," I reminded her.

"Okay, Mom," she smiled, "thanks for doing this."

Shift: It's something we all have to learn. I just hope that I have taught her to shift well. I think I have. I know the kind of person she has become. She is smart and confident. She is tenacious and strong despite her slight appearance. She is beautiful inside and out. I love my Emily more than she'll ever know. I love her kindness and gentle spirit, and I know that her ability to shift will grow stronger as she drives down the road of life.

Chapter 9

UNsettled

Through Eva's Eyes

Life's constant shifting is like a sudden sandstorm, which rises out of nowhere and transforms our orderly world into chaos. A few grains of sand are tolerable; they can be swept up or swept under the bed or ignored. A sandstorm, on the other hand, demands immediate attention—maybe even a bulldozer. I don't own a bulldozer, only a tractor. I wanted to bulldoze Aaron right out of our lives forever, but that didn't appear to be an option at the moment.

After the meeting, I looked at my devastated daughter as she sat at the table in her wheelchair with tears streaming down her cheeks, and I wanted to do more than just bulldoze Aaron. I wanted to bury him alive! Dreadful images of his demise funnel-clouded through my brain, leaving angry grains of sand in every crease and crevasse.

I sat at the table next to Jessica, crying my share of tears. Eva broke away from playing school with Aunt Emily and brought us paper towels from the kitchen. She climbed on my lap, and I held her close and hugged her—no words necessary. I didn't have any words. Jessica handed me her wedding ring. Eva noticed the exchange, and great sadness shadowed her three-year-old face. Such sorrow should never dim a three-year-old face. It just shouldn't happen. Three-year-olds are meant to be happy and carefree, not sad and brooding.

I can only imagine what was going through Eva's mind as she cuddled on my lap. She just witnessed her father storm out of the house without her mother or her. Now, her crying mother has removed her wedding ring. This little child's life was torn apart again in an instant. Yes, she had all of us to comfort her, but words escaped me at the moment. How could she comprehend what was happening to her mommy and daddy? She must have been terrified, wondering what would happen to her. I held her tight, buried my tear-stained face in her hair, and prayed a silent prayer for protection over her.

"Come on, Eva," Emily coaxed Eva off my lap. "Let's go play school."

Thankfully, Eva's sadness was replaced quickly with joy. Eva's eyes lit up with the promise of putting Aunt Emily in the time-out the chair again—Eva's favorite thing to do.

"You better behave, Aunt Emily, or you're going straight to the principal's office..." Eva's voice trailed off as they made their way to Eva's classroom.

Those eyes! Those beautiful blue eyes, so much like her mother's. When I looked at Eva's eyes, I saw the little girl that Jessica was, the little girl that loved to play school and grew up to be a schoolteacher. I saw the little girl that put her teddy bear named Aaron (of course) in the time out chair over and over again: the little girl that did flips and cartwheels almost every day of her life. In this way, Eva was just like her mommy. She was a cartwheel queen and loved her trampoline. Eva had the body of a gymnast, too, and would have lived at the gym if we let her.

Jess, so much like Eva, literally grew up in a gym with Romanian coaches named Gregory and Luba, who were going to make her a star athlete. My daughter, the gymnast. Yes, I admit it, I was a gymnastics mom. No, I was not like the dance moms you see on TV now, not outwardly anyway. Inwardly, I longed to watch my daughter compete in the Olympics. I still think she could have, but she became a diver. She was good. Jessica was good at most sports, a natural athlete. Jessica was in great shape, so healthy, so energetic, so...alive! So, why? Why, God? Why?

That's too simplistic, isn't it—cliché. Crying out to God over and over again as if He'll answer. Cliché or not, I hurt, and I'm angry, and I don't understand His reasoning—His purpose in doing this to my daughter!

The Farm

December 2016

Where's my twine? I'm not done spinning this yarn. I've just begun. Let's see, where was I? That's right; I was smelling the Juicy Fruit gum back when I was three and hoping no one would tell me that my mommy went to the store. I can't undo what happened to me, nor can I undo what happened to Jess. I can't even get a "redo." All I can do is write and hope that this story might touch someone.

Eva's three. I'm thinking of this as I'm typing. *Three years old and her life is being thrown into turmoil!* The world is full of such promise at three. I'm lost now. Lost in thought. It's getting cloudy. The sunny spot on the ground is long gone, and my behind is numb. I should go back inside and check on Jessica. She's probably done with her nap by now and wants to pee. That's what she seems to do these days—nap and pee.

It wasn't always like this, although it seems the days of Jessica calling me on the phone just to check in and give me an Eva update are long gone. So are the days of going and volunteering in her classroom full of snot-nosed first graders who could not comprehend that Jessica had a mommy. As we all know, first-grade teachers live at the school and have no life outside of elaborate bulletin boards and classrooms full of stick figures in fields of crayon flowers.

I remember one day when I volunteered and ate lunch with Jessica's class. The main topic of conversation was about birthdays and teeth—losing teeth—to be exact. Tooth Fairy comparisons were topping the list. I don't think any of the children at my table could relate to my tooth fairy's enormous payout of five cents. One thing I did learn from my lunch table discussions was that Jessica, "Mrs. R," was loved by all her students. Of course, I had to write a story about her.

Chapter 10

UNruly

Mrs. R

As bits of his peanut butter and jelly sandwich sprayed from his mouth landing precariously close to my lunch plate, seven-year-old Joe said, " Mrs. R was made in the 1980s."

"She was 'bornded' on the same day as me," Shayla chimed in, "on number 23. I was bornded on the number 23 too, but in February, and Mrs. R was bornded on the number 23 in March." She grinned at me, revealing a gaping hole where two teeth used to be. Indeed, most of my lunch table companions were missing at least two teeth.

"Were you there when Mrs. R was bornded?" Jacob asked.

"I remember it well," I replied as pictures of the delivery room danced in my head. Mrs. R was refusing to be born, so the nurse was straddling me, pushing on my belly as a last-ditch effort before rushing me to surgery for a C-section. Luckily, the nurse's Herculean efforts paid off, and Mrs. R was born; only back then, her name wasn't Mrs. R; it was Jessica. "I'm Mrs. R's mommy," I explained. "So, I was there when she was born."

"Mrs. R has a mommy!" Josh exclaimed.

Some of the more worldly children at my table patiently explained to Josh that everyone has a mommy—even Mrs. R.

The reason we were all discussing Mrs. R's birthday is that she had just celebrated her twenty-fifth birthday a few days before. In the world of seven-year-olds, birthdays are ranked first in the top ten most important life events, followed closely by losing teeth.

"So," I asked my table of munchkins, "can anyone tell me where all your teeth went?"

"The 'toof' fairy took mine," Elizabeth yelled from the end of the table. Even though she was shouting, I was finding it hard to hear her over the chatter of the surrounding lunch tables. It didn't help matters when they all started talking at once:

"I got five."

"Once...I lost three..."

"The tooth fairy left me..."

"Dollars..."

"Teeth...a note..."

"At once..."

"When I fell off my bicycle."

As the children clambered for my attention, I glanced over at Jessica, who was sitting at another table eating lunch with the rest of her class. The chatter going on at her table was as lively as mine. I had to smile as I observed the adoring faces of the children surrounding my daughter. It seems like only yesterday; she was sitting on the floor of her bedroom with all her stuffed animals surrounding her.

I remember vividly one particular day: she was telling her furry kindergarten class the story of Goldilocks and the Three Bears. She couldn't have been more than five herself; in fact, I think she was still in preschool. She had set up a makeshift chalkboard (a piece of cardboard), and she was holding her pointer (a stick from our yard).

By her side, she had a box of stickers (a must-have for all kindergarten teachers). As she told the story, she periodically pointed to the invisible scenes on her chalkboard while asking questions of her well-behaved students.

I noticed that most of her stuffed animals were covered in "great job" stickers—all except one. Then, I discovered why. I didn't know that Jessica was aware of my presence in the doorway until she turned to the "stickerless" dog and sternly informed him that the principal was here to get him. I took that as my cue and entered the classroom.

"Miss Jessica," I said in my dour principal voice, "do you have a student who is misbehaving?"

"Yes," she replied. "Will you please take Aaron to the office and call his mother? Tell her that Aaron keeps interrupting our story."

"I will," I said gruffly as I took Aaron by the paw and escorted him out of the room.

I still marvel at the fact that she has never wavered from her dream of becoming a teacher. She would come home from school and play school. Even on weekends, she would play school. In fact, the neighborhood kids would send their stuffed animals to Jessica's school. Jessica didn't become a teacher. Jessica was bornded a teacher!

Since then, I have had the privilege of volunteering in her class (and I didn't even have to play the part of the gruff principal). That day, as we were walking to the lunchroom, I noticed how happy all her students were. They didn't walk to the lunchroom, they bounced, hopped, skipped, spun, and laughed. They weren't misbehaving in line; it was just a happy line.

I commented to Jessica that they were a merry bunch. She laughed and said that she'd been told by a lot of teachers that her class had become transformed since she took over. The previous teacher became ill and had to retire in the middle of the school year.

Mrs. R didn't fly in like Super Woman, and she didn't even wear a cape, but to her students, she was a hero. Her classroom was a place of joy where the children felt safe and loved. She's my hero, too. She has grown into a beautiful, kind woman whom I have the honor of calling my daughter.

We were getting up from our lunchroom table when I heard a voice at my side, "Are you Mrs. R's mommy?" I looked in the direction of the tiny voice and saw a small child who must have been about five. "I want to be in her class when I grow up," the voice continued, "because she is the 'bestest' teacher in the whole school!"

Most of us can point to that one teacher that had a profound impact on our lives. I know Mrs. R's students will remember her for years to come. She may even be the "bestest teacher in the whole world" to that one child who just needed someone to care. Perhaps Kyle summed it up best as I sat next to him during reading instruction. "Before Mrs. R came, my reading was broken," he confessed. Then he grinned proudly and pronounced, "But, she is helping me fix it. She is fixing all my broken spots."

Reflection

Jessica's life as a teacher, her lifelong dream, has been diminished for now to volunteering. She once taught with me by her side, always by her side. I'm Jessica's sidekick now, and sometimes I cry about it. Sometimes I just burst into tears because I don't want to be my daughter's sidekick. I don't want to be her everything anymore. I did that already. You hear me, God? I did that already! I *was* her everything when she was an infant and a toddler and a first-grader. I did the mommy thing already.

Jessica says she'll teach again. Although she also says that volunteering is better than teaching because she doesn't have to deal with the lesson plans and all the other BS that's required of teachers these days. Jessica says one day she'll walk into the classroom again. Jessica has a fantastic attitude. She calls her husband an asshole and moves on. She doesn't dwell or wallow as I do now. No, Jessica picks up the pieces of her life and smiles and laughs because maybe, just maybe she knows how quickly life can be taken from us. She knows that life shouldn't be wasted on wallowing because it only takes a second to have everything change.

That's what happened. It was one second. One second Jessica was running down her quiet neighborhood street at dawn, and the next second she was having a seizure in the middle of the road. Jack and I weren't in town because it was a holiday, and we decided to go away for a long weekend. Jessica had the day off from school, which is why she decided to go for a run. I got the call from Aaron as we were heading out for a day of exploring The Villages with my sister.

Memorial Hospital

October 2015

"What? What?" I kept saying it over and over again because I couldn't believe my ears.

"It's Jessica..." Aaron managed to choke out through his sobs. "She's been taken to the hospital...I don't know. A guy found her in the middle of the road."

"Drive home!" I yelled at Jack.

"What's going on?" Jack asked.

"It's Jessica," I answered.

Bewilderment shrouded both our faces now. We flagged down my sister in the car in front of us.

"We have to go home. Jessica is in the hospital," I said.

"What?" My sister and brother-in-law exclaimed in unison.

"I don't know what's wrong," I said. "Someone found her on the road."

We knew very little as we took the three-hour drive back home. Bits and pieces of information flooded in via phone calls from Aaron. Three hospitals. Seizures. Breathing tube. Unconscious. Emergency surgery on her brain.

I called my sister's cell phone. "You better come now," I managed to choke out.

I cried as my sister listened silently on the other end of the line. No, I didn't just cry. I wailed. No words are adequate to describe the misery.

My sister just said, "Okay, we're coming." Then I guess she hung up.

I don't know how Jack drove. Not one word was spoken between us. Our daughter Lucy was in the backseat. I could hear her quietly weeping. Her sounds were awful as she tried to mute them—as if keeping them at bay would make things less real.

I called Emily. No answer. Voicemail. *Damn!*

Silence shrouded our car except for Lucy's heart-wrenching sobs. By the time we reached the hospital, there were already about fifty people overflowing from the surgery waiting room. Emily was there, thank God. She ran to us. We all held on to each other—Emily, Lucy, Jack, and I. We just held on for a long time, each lost in our private misery.

We found Aaron in the sea of people. He spotted us, and we made our way out to the front of the hospital.

"She's in surgery," he said flatly.

No, duh, I thought to myself as I tried desperately to pull myself together and ask an intelligent question.

"What happened?" It's all I could muster.

"They took her to the first hospital and thought it was a trauma case since she was on the road jogging (maybe hit by a car). The doctors called ahead to the second hospital, and they transferred her there, where the trauma team was waiting. The trauma doctor was the one who said he didn't believe this was trauma and sent her here where the brain surgeon is on duty.

The surgeon said she had a brain aneurysm that ruptured. She has two more that he has to coil, so they don't burst." Aaron's matter-of-fact report seemed surreal to me. It was as if he were talking about a stranger, not his wife. There was no emotion in his account.

None of this was making any sense to me. I couldn't comprehend my healthy twenty-nine-year-old daughter suffering from something usually associated with someone much older. It didn't matter, though, because it happened to her, and now she was in surgery.

"How bad?" I asked.

"Bad," Aaron said. "She has a 50/50 chance of making it through this surgery to stop the bleeding. Then, she'll need more surgeries for the coils."

"Coils?" I asked. "What's that?"

"Something the doctor does to the other two aneurysms to keep them from bursting," Aaron explained.

I didn't really understand what he was saying, but I didn't want to push it at that moment.

Aaron left then and walked to the curb, sat down, and put his head in his hands.

Jack sat next to him. A little over a year later, after Aaron's goodwill drop off at our house, Jack decided he should tell me what Aaron was mumbling into his hands the day his wife almost died.

Aaron's grief was evident, but it wasn't for Jess. He was sobbing alright, but his words spoke louder than his actions and painted a more accurate picture of the real Aaron.

As Jack sat on the curb next to Aaron, he heard his words loud and clear. "I can't believe this is happening to me!"

Aaron wasn't thinking about Jess, and Aaron wasn't thinking about Eva either. Aaron was only thinking about himself.

Eva wasn't at the hospital. She was in the care of her grandma, Anne. Eva never came to Memorial Hospital. She never came to Holy Cross Hospital, but I'm getting ahead of myself now.

Our lives changed forever when the horror happened to Jess. The ball of twine that was all our lives grew prodigiously overnight, it seems. Friends quickly became family, and we were blessed to be surrounded by a group of believers who lifted us all in prayer.

While Jess had tubes coming out of every orifice in her body and machines monitored her brain activity and swelling, we prayed. While machines breathed for her, circulated her blood, helped her heartbeat, emptied her bladder, fed her fluids, and gave her drugs, we prayed. Prayer was all we had because the doctors were doing everything in their power to keep Jess alive, and they were not giving us hope in a medical miracle. They were not miracle workers. There was only one miracle worker I knew, and I prayed to Him as I've never prayed before.

I don't think we would have made it through any of this without our friends and family and their constant prayers. They helped us plan a prayer vigil in the field outside the hospital. By then, the entire hospital knew about Jessica, and many said they were praying for us.

Hundreds attended the vigil, including many people from the hospital staff.

The turnout was astonishing with Jess and Aaron's church friends, our friends, family, Jess's coworkers, and Jack's coworkers all in attendance. There were too many people for me to count. It was a beautiful ceremony with the candlelight illuminating the entire field! I wish with all my heart that Jess could have seen the outpouring of support for her.

Unfortunately, Eva wasn't among the praying. Her father thought it best that she stay at home with her grandmother. But I'm getting ahead of myself again.

My way of coping with life is to write. I have always written journals and stories ever since I can remember. So, it was only fitting that I'd take on the role of keeping everyone informed of Jessica's progress through an online journal that keeps people up to date on loved ones who are sick. This way, people can check on someone without disturbing the family with constant phone calls. The website is aptly named CaringBridge. It acts as a bridge for families and friends who care about the individual and want to keep themselves informed.

Reflection

I'm glad I took on the role of the CaringBridge writer because it helped me sort out my feelings and was my public way of praying for Jess. I wanted to honor God through all of the struggles because I wanted people to see faith in action.

Chapter 11

UNfaltering

The Farm

December 2016

The donkeys start braying. They're hungry. I'm shirking my farmer duties in the hopes of stealing precious time for writing. Who am I kidding? There's no time for writing—no time for thought streams. There are plenty of streams that need tending to right now: streams of clothes waiting patiently by the washer, streams of dishes cascading into the sink, streams of dirt streaking the tile floor...streams of tears running down my face.

Time to stop writing and feed the brayers, barkers, meowers, and cock-a-doodle-dooers. No time to write. Not today.

I try to "unperch." I can't. Maybe it's because my knees are frozen in place, even in this heat. Perhaps I cannot unperch because the will just isn't there. The braying tugs me. The laundry cries loud enough for me to cover my ears. I don't want to pay attention to any of it. I don't want anything or anyone to expect me to pay attention. I don't want to be responsible. Does anyone get that? "Leave me alone!" I shout into the nothingness. "Let me be!" I yell. I'm losing it. My fingers type, losing it—big time.

It's ok to lose it today, though, because it is my birthday. Birthdays close to Christmas may be short on

88

presents, but they tend to have lots of presence. There are lots of people in the house today. Jack is still home from school on his politically correct winter break. Lucy is home too and currently in the kitchen trying to bring herself to torture and kill a live lobster in boiling water (for my birthday dinner).

Emily is home on vacation as well, most likely caring for Jessica right now as I have flown the coop to the pasture to write. I'm assuming no one is missing me—at least no one with two legs. The four-legged ones are still loudly telling me that supper is late. Oh well, they'll just have to wait a little longer. I'm on a roll here.

Where was I? That's right; I was losing it. I think I was yelling at God.

As Jessica would say, "Mom, you lost it a long time ago." Jessica has a way with words. Her sharp wit is still intact, perhaps even more so now that her filter is gone. Aaron is often the brunt of Jessica's jokes. When someone asks her how she's doing, she usually holds up her left hand and says, "Great! Look how well I can lift my hand now that it's so much lighter without that damn ring!"

A year ago, she couldn't move that hand at all. A year ago, she couldn't speak. A year ago, I stood by her hospital bed, singing soft lullabies to the beat of 13 dripping IV tubes and the drumming of the respirator. A year ago, I would never have guessed that Jessica would be holding up her ringless left hand and flipping Aaron the bird.

A year ago, Emily and I carried blow-up mattresses into the area of the ICU waiting room that our family and friends commandeered. It was clear that we weren't going anywhere, despite the very loud protestations of the security guard.

In short order, two recliners, blankets, and pillows arrived in the waiting room courtesy of the president of the hospital board of directors. Along with the recliners, we received a handful of free meal tickets for the cafeteria. It seemed everyone at the hospital knew about Jessica, and everyone, all the way to the top, was pulling for her.

A year ago, I stopped writing. Well, I still wrote, but it was updates on CaringBridge. I tried to write the updates with honesty and insight. Sometimes I was able to accomplish a mediocre update, but mostly I was typing with numb fingers pecking out the ramblings of a mostly numb brain.

I always tried to be thoughtful about what I wrote on CaringBridge. I knew that people wanted to be filled with hope. I wanted to be filled with hope. I'd think: *What am I going to say? Should I tell everyone that the doctors are giving us little if any, hope? Should I talk about the conversation with Jessica's nurse, who was encouraging us to turn off the respirator? Should I talk about the "fact" that Jessica was most likely going to die or, if she survived, was going to require round-the-clock skilled nursing, aka a nursing home? Should I tell everyone that she had a stroke on top of the brain bleeds and was paralyzed now on her left side? Should I express the impossible to quell emotions that bombard me every day?*

I cannot close the Pandora Box of emotions once they come crashing out. I ride the waves of sadness and despair every day far more often than the wave of hope. Sorrow and hopelessness wash over me when I hold Jess's hand, and there is no response. They sweep me away when I look at the shaking heads of the doctors every morning during rounds. I ride the desperation wave at least several times a day. The thing about brain aneurysms is that they don't often bring waves of hope. Brain aneurysms crash onto shore as a tsunami, and they tend to destroy everything in their wake.

"Not this time," I shout to the brain aneurysm tsunami. "NO! You will *not* take my daughter. Not on my watch." I knew I had to let go of the tsunami and ride the hope wave, so I wrote hope in CaringBridge posts, and I tried to pour that hope into my heart.

I wrote about God and how He was healing our daughter. I wrote about the expectancy of God's promise. I wrote about unwavering faith because I wanted to convince myself that my faith would not falter. I tried to "fake it until you make it."

I did believe, but I also doubted. Sometimes, I wrote about my doubts. I also wrote about how Jack fell asleep at the red light on the way to the hospital or how none of us slept for days on end.

Jack, Emily, Jess's aunts and uncles, and I took shifts at the hospital so that Jess would never be alone. Often, I took a night shift and then slept in the ICU waiting room while someone else took the day shift.

Jack often took night shifts and then went to work the next day on no sleep at all. Friends and family made schedules for feeding those of us who lived at the hospital.

Occasionally, someone would volunteer to stay with Jess, and I'd leave to go home and shower, but I always returned as soon as I could just in case a finger moved or, the miracle of all miracles, Jess awoke. My hope wave was still cresting, and every day I tried to catch it.

I tried to articulate our family's daily struggles on CaringBridge. No matter how hard I tried, though, I had difficulty capturing the realness of the situation. I couldn't convey the awfulness of it all. I couldn't tell everyone that it appeared hopeless—at least from the doctors' perspective.

Through the darkest of days, our family remained prayerful. I knew Jess was hanging on by a thread, but I found hope in the movement of a finger and the fluttering of an eyelid. I found hope in the removal of one more IV bag. I found hope in rainbows and the dawning of every new day. I found hope in Jessica's fighting spirit. I found hope in God—the ultimate healer.

Chapter 12

UNimaginable

Day 11

November 6, 2015

Psalm 30 speaks of the blessedness of answered prayer. I picked two verses from Psalm 30 that seem to fit right now: "...Weeping may endure for a night, but joy cometh in the morning" (Ps 30:5 KJV). "Thou hast turned for me my mourning into dancing..." (Ps 30:11).

I wasn't dancing yet. Far from it. I wept all night that night. I wept for my vibrant, beautiful baby girl and her baby girl. I wept for my children and my husband. I wept for our extended family and friends who are all struggling too. I wept for Jessica's adorable students in her first-grade class. I wept and wept. There is no describing the kind of weeping I experienced that night.

But joy did come that morning when I heard that we could proceed with Jessica's tracheotomy. I never thought in a million years that I would be joyful over my daughter getting a breathing tube, but it is better than a ventilator, and she would be more comfortable.

It was Day 11, and the surgery was scheduled for 3:00. I was sitting by her side, watching her rest quietly and listening to the song, "Christ Alone Cornerstone." I couldn't help but feel His presence "right here right now." I knew it was going to be a long road ahead. Jessica would go to a long-term care facility that specialized in traumatic brain injury. I was hopeful for her future. I was hopeful for the future of her family because I knew that God was shining his favor on us.

I was thankful that so many loving doctors and nurses surrounded her. I was so grateful for the friends and family that surrounded our family. I have watched many families come through the ICU waiting room, some so very alone. I can honestly say that our family and friends continued to be a shining example of strength and dignity. Jessica was indeed clothed in strength and dignity, and I had every confidence that she would laugh in the days to come.

Day 14

November 9, 2015

I couldn't believe how much our lives changed in two weeks. I remember the last conversation I had with Jess about her plans for the four day weekend. Of course, she was planning to take Eva to the park and then go into her classroom and catch up on some work. Her dedication to her family and her first-grade class was always evident in everything she did. God, how I missed hearing her voice and seeing her smile.

Never in a million years did I ever think that I'd be writing updates on how she's breathing! But there I was sitting at the keyboard. And I was writing about how my vibrant, beautiful, dedicated, strong daughter was breathing on her own now. It was so heart wrenching because we all just wanted Jessica to sit up and say something simple like, "Where am I?" or "What happened?"

As each day passed, I realized that all our lives had been forever altered, and I was in the depths of despair. But I wouldn't stay there. I couldn't stay there. I would not stay there! As hard as it was, I knew I must reach into my soul and find the strength and the peace that surpasses all understanding. I knew that is what Jessica would want, and I knew that is what she needed.

She needed our love and our strength. She needed to know that she was safe and that we would never leave her side. I looked again at the pictures of Jess and Aaron's church family gathered around Aaron praying. It was such a moving tribute to both of them. Those pictures spoke volumes about the support that surrounded our family.

At last, she was breathing without the assistance of the ventilator. That was an excellent sign. She was running a fever, which was frequently seen in brain trauma, but they were keeping a close eye on that. She was moving her right arm, purposefully. When I sang to her, she moved her head in my direction. I don't know if it was because she wanted me to stop singing or to keep it up.

The following weekend, we attended an outside wedding. It was pouring on our way there, and we thought for sure that the wedding would be moved inside. However, we were told to wait to see if the rain let up. I was standing with another friend whose husband was battling cancer. We were talking about our struggles, and I said to her that if the rain lets up, we should ask God to send us a rainbow.

Well, the rain did stop, and we were ushered to our seats. Just as the bride arrived, a rainbow appeared over the trees. The rain started again within minutes of the end of the ceremony. Later, I asked my friend if she saw the rainbow. She said yes, and there were actually two of them!

Day 19

Lullaby

November 14, 2015

Sometimes I sang lullabies to my sleeping daughter just as I did when I rocked her in my arms some 29 years before. How I wanted to scoop her up again and hold her close so she could feel my heartbeat in rhythm with hers. It was like I had my baby back all over again. I had to observe her and learn what she needed using instinct, just like when she was an infant. I prayed to God to give me the strength to hold her again and the courage to fight for her and with her. I looked forward to our journey together, especially to the day when she could hold her baby again. Meanwhile, I just kept singing her lullabies.

Reflection

Looking back now, I remember one terrible night when Jess just kept thrashing and moaning, and I didn't know what to do to soothe her. Finally, out of desperation, I called the nurse, and she asked me if I had changed her diaper. It never occurred to me that I should check my grown daughter's diaper! The nurse checked it for me and said she believed that was the problem. After she changed her, Jess fell fast asleep. I couldn't help but think my daughter was a newborn all over again, and I was a new mother all over again. I just hoped I was up to the task.

Chapter 13

UNresponsive

The Farm

December 2016

Reflecting over the months in the hospitals with Jess, I can't help but remember that awful ambulance ride from south Florida to north Florida. For over seven hours, I rode shotgun as my comatose daughter was lying on a stretcher, being kept alive and comfortable behind me. I cannot recall the thoughts running through my brain that day, but I can still feel the emotions: sadness, regret, hope, and apprehension. All were swimming through my consciousness as the ambulance meandered through the endless traffic, and the driver remained utterly silent. Anger, too, reared its ugly head as I thought about Aaron and the fact that it wasn't him riding shotgun in the ambulance, but I'm getting ahead of myself again.

Chapter 14

UNreal

Holy Cross Hospital

I sat in the front of the ambulance with the non-communicative driver while Jess rode on the stretcher in the back with an attendant taking her vitals every fifteen minutes. Paramedic number two was much chattier than paramedic number one. Number two talked to Jessica the entire time, despite the fact that she had been heavily sedated for the trip. I guess paramedic number two felt that it was more productive talking to Jess than his partner, who never uttered a single word during the seven and half hour trek.

I finally gave up after an hour of futile attempts at learning the driver's name. I didn't bother to ask the name of the paramedic caring for Jess. I was unable to talk to paramedic number two because of the divider between the passenger seat and the back section.

The extent of my interactions with the paramedics for that day consisted of a few words between me and paramedic number two. That was when I got out of the ambulance to use the bathroom at a convenience store. "How's she doing?"

"Fine," replied number two. "Her vitals have been stable the entire time so far."

I didn't know where Aaron or Sherry, Jess's friend from church, were since they appeared to take a different route than the ambulance. I thought about calling Aaron just to let him know that his wife was fine, but I figured he'd call me if he wanted to know how Jess was doing. I was still more than a little perturbed that it was me riding in the ambulance instead of him. I could have driven his truck or my car. He could have taken my car back. I was planning on staying at Holy Cross Hospital with Jess, so I didn't need a vehicle.

I thought it was strange that Sherry did not ride with Aaron in his car, but she later confided that her husband requested they go in separate cars. What was that all about? I wondered but never pursued that line of questioning with Sherry. I didn't know her that well and didn't feel it was my place to ask.

It took the ambulance seven and a half hours, three of them in bumper-to-bumper rush-hour traffic, to finally arrive at Holy Cross Hospital. While the paramedics were wheeling Jessica into her new digs, I scanned the parking lot for signs of Aaron or Sherry. They were nowhere in sight. *That's weird*, I thought, *they should have gotten here before us.*

I had to sign all of Jessica's admission papers, leaving lots of blanks with an explanation to the admission's clerk that Jess's husband would be here any minute to complete the forms. Aaron's arrival didn't happen before the clerk gave up hope. As the clerk started closing up shop, he admonished me to make sure Aaron came in early in the morning to complete the forms. The clerk seemed to be questioning whether Aaron really existed. I was beginning to wonder the same thing!

After about an hour, Aaron called me. A nurse and I were in Jess's room, getting her settled when my phone rang. Imagine my surprise when Aaron said he and Sherry were at the mall and wanted to know what I wanted for dinner. To say I was speechless is an understatement. I don't remember quite what I said, but I'm sure it had nothing to do with what I wanted for dinner. I'm certain the nurse was wondering with whom I was speaking by the time I disconnected the call.

"That was Jess's husband," I explained. "He wanted to know what I want for dinner. He's at the mall."

The nurse looked as dumbfounded as I felt. Her expression mirrored my contempt for Aaron at that moment. "He's at the mall? Why?"

"I don't know," I said with a tinge of sarcasm. "Doesn't everyone go to the mall when their spouse is being transferred from one hospital to another via ambulance?"

After our brief exchange, the nurse and I busied ourselves with Jess. Jess fell asleep quickly. The nurse provided some sheets, blankets, and a pillow for the pull-out bed next to Jess's bed. I made the bed and promptly fell asleep next to Jess.

I don't know how much time elapsed before Aaron and Sherry arrived, but I was sound asleep and in no mood for dinner. Sherry had a lot of shopping bags in tow and was very excited to show me all the items she purchased for Jess's hospital stay: bras, panties, PJ's, and comfortable clothes. I imagined that Sherry must have called Aaron to say that she was going to stop off at the mall to get some items for Jess, and he said he'd meet her there.

I don't think this was a pre-planned stop, or one of them would have mentioned it to me before the long ride. I didn't blame Sherry for Aaron's disregard for his wife. I honestly felt that Sherry's heart was in the right place. I didn't know what to think about Aaron's heart at that moment. The two of them didn't stay long at the hospital since Jess was sleeping, and I was clearly exhausted. Soon, they were off to the hotel for a good night's sleep. Of course, they had to be well rested for the long trip back home the next day.

Reflection

Aaron was very instrumental in the decision to have Jess evaluated for Holy Cross Rehabilitation. He insisted that Jess belonged somewhere where there would be an opportunity for her to receive the best rehab possible. He scoured the state for the right hospital and hounded them until they sent a nurse to evaluate Jess. I am thankful that Aaron was so persistent because the alternative for Jess would have been a mediocre local rehab facility that primarily provided a bed, a nursing staff, and a few OT and PT therapists.

Holy Cross, on the other hand, provided extensive inpatient care with state-of-the-art equipment and a team of doctors and therapists that continually monitored patient progress. Holy Cross was very particular about the patients they took and frequently turned people away who they thought had little to no ability to meet the milestones in each progressive level. Based on the fact that Jess's communication was limited to blinking once for yes and twice for no, we were not very optimistic that the evaluation would go well.

The nurse from Holy Cross was a pleasant gentleman who told us upfront that he didn't think Jess would qualify even for the minimally conscious unit. He started his evaluation by testing Jess's reflexes in her feet and moved to her hands. He talked to her the entire time, asking her to blink if she could hear him. She didn't. The fact that Jess still had a tracheostomy (a hole with a tube in her windpipe) was another strike against her being accepted into Holy Cross.

As the nurse explained, they don't like to take such medically challenged patients. Jess was medically challenged on many levels with several of her vital systems still mechanically monitored and her level of brain function completely uncertain. Often, the nurses have to tell people to wait until the patient has made more progress. That is what we fully expected to hear from the Holy Cross nurse.

I truly believe that had it not been for Aaron's dogged persistence and constant contact with the evaluating nurse, Jess would have been rejected for the minimally conscious unit. The nurse told me that he was making his decision based on the outpouring of support and love of Jess's family since it is imperative that the family be involved in the patient's rehab. He said that if anyone had at making it, it would be Jess strictly because she had so many people who cared about her.

The nurse came back to the hospital three times to meet with us, and each time he told us that he's never seen so many people praying for one patient. However, he reminded us, if Jess didn't make significant progress within the first three weeks, then she would be released with the promise that they'd take her back when she was ready to graduate from the minimally conscious level.

Chapter 15

UNconcerned

When Jessica arrived at Holy Cross Hospital, she was considered to be in a pre-emergent state. In other words, she wasn't breathing without the tracheostomy tube. She wasn't talking, and she wasn't moving any of her limbs or even fully opening her eyes. Jessica was blinking once for yes and twice for no. That was about it, but we kept telling the doctors that she was still far too sedated, mostly from pain medication, to show them what she could do. The doctors at Holy Cross Hospital finally listened to us and started weening Jessica off the pain medicine.

Slowly, Jessica started emerging as they call it at Holy Cross Hospital. The emerging stage was not an easy one—not for Jessica and not for me. It started with Jessica's right leg and arm in constant motion, like a one-legged perpetual marching soldier. In unison, non-stop, her right leg and arm went up and down as if someone were winding and rewinding a giant spring-loaded key in Jessica's back. Up and down—up and down.

The marching went on day and night with no end in sight! I couldn't sleep because Jessica was so strong that she was practically propelling herself out of the top of her bed with each leg movement. I had to be constantly vigilant to prevent Jess from injuring herself by falling out of bed. I'd pull her down, and her right quad would push her up over and over again. It was exhausting.

The nightly wrestling matches went on well into the wee hours of the morning. Often, I'd still be awake when the nurse came into the room at 3 a.m. with the schedule for the day. During the first early morning delivery, the nurse tried to sneak in without disturbing us. She didn't know I was awake and was so startled when I said hello that she practically jumped out of her shoes.

The next two nights, she expected me to be awake because Jess showed no signs of slowing her marching rhythm. By the fourth night, it became evident that I could not continue the non-stop vigilance. Short of chaining Jess to the bed, there had to be some way to contain her. "Net bed" were the words that the staff kept bantering about.

They told me that the only way to keep Jessica safe was to put her in a net bed. I didn't know at the time why the staff dreaded the net bed, but I knew I needed to sleep, and Jess needed to be safe as she thrashed about, so I said, "Bring in the dreaded net bed."

Day 24

November 19, 2015

A tough time for me was seeing the frustration and confusion that accompanied Jess's recovery. As she "emerged" and explored her environment, she was doing many things that you'd expect from a baby. It was as if the world were opening up to her all at once, and she didn't quite know what to make of it or how to respond to it.

Everyone kept commenting on how strong Jess was, and the "propelling herself off the bed" maneuver proved she was not only strong but cunning. The new net bed was like a giant pack and play. I don't believe Jessica liked it much. One night, she started to get agitated around 6 p.m. and worked herself into a frenzy for about five hours.

It was so hard for me to watch this. I couldn't figure out what was wrong, and she couldn't tell me—much like an infant. All my motherly instincts failed me, and I could not make her comfortable no matter what I did. I finally just broke down and started crying at her bedside. She looked over at me and blew me a kiss. Of course, that made me cry more.

I wished I could take this pain, frustration, and agitation away from her. I wished I could put her in a car seat and drive her around the block a million times (she always fell asleep in the car). I wished so many things for my daughter. I wished that she could hold her baby girl in her arms. I wished that she could use the damn marker on the whiteboard of her classroom instead of trying to draw a line on the therapist's paper. I wished she would say, "Hey, Mom, do you want to go to the beach this weekend?" Instead, I pushed her around in her wheelchair!

I was so tired. When I had a moment to reflect on how tired I was, I got scared that I wouldn't be able to see her through this. I never signed up for this. I never signed up for changing the diaper of my grown child. God, it was so hard! She blew me another kiss when she saw me crying as I typed this.

Okay, enough of my hissy fit. I would be remiss if I didn't mention how thankful I was for the staff of Holy Cross Hospital and their tremendous support and infinite patience with all my questions. I have to remember that this emerging stage of recovery was very tough but necessary. It was difficult because, as her brain "woke up" and reconnected, all her senses started flooding her at once.

Imagine a brutal battle where you are stuck in a foxhole with everyone around you shooting at you. Only, they're not shooting bullets. They're shooting sound, touch, smells, taste, and sights, and you have no way to filter the projectiles bombarding your brain. You can't tell them to stop shooting at you because you cannot talk. The only way your body knows how to deal with the deluge is to flood itself with something soothing, like marching in place or rocking back and forth.

I have to remember that this level of frustration Jess was feeling was a good sign. And, through all of this, I had to remember the promise of the rainbows. I had to know that God was going to give both Jessica and me the strength to endure. "But they that wait upon the LORD shall renew their strength; they shall mount up with wings as eagles; they shall run, and not be weary; and they shall walk, and not faint" (Isa. 40:31).

By the time the net bed arrived, I was delirious from lack of sleep, and Jessica was still marching to the beat of the one-sided drummer in her head. I don't know how she endured the marching—she even marched in her sleep. The doctors had finally found a drug concoction to induce a few hours of sleep for Jessica, but the zip-up net bed terrified her. Not even the drugs calmed her the first few nights in the net bed.

My makeshift bed, a pull-out couch with no padding to speak of, was right next to Jessica's net bed. I'd hear her moaning and thrashing all night long, and my heart would break over and over again because I was helpless to relieve her anxiety. A broken heart—that's what I had. At the time, I didn't realize how broken my heart truly was!

So, Jessica and I endured the vile net bed for at least three days and nights until it became as much a permanent fixture in the hospital room as the IV poles and custom wheelchair.

After about two weeks, Jess was given a break from therapy so we could visit the wheelchair room. What a great place. I kept thinking that I'd love to work in the wheelchair room because I love to tinker, build, and fix things. The purpose of the visit was to build a wheelchair that was just perfect for Jess. The first step was to interview Jess and me.

"Does she sit up without assistance?"

"No."

"Does she fall over when sitting up?"

"Yes."

"Does she have the use of both hands?"

"No. Her left hand and arm are paralyzed."

"Is she aware of where she is in space?"

"I don't know what that means."

"Can she manipulate objects?"

"Only objects that are on her right side because she has very minimal peripheral vision out of her left eye and cannot move her left arm."

"How does she communicate?"

"She can talk a little bit, although she has difficulty putting her thoughts together. She kisses everyone when she is happy."

"Can she stand?"

"In a standing machine."

"Can she move her legs?"

"Her right leg only."

"Can she bend both legs?"

"Yes."

"Can she keep her head up?"

"Yes."

"How long?"

"I don't know."

The questions went on for about 20 minutes. I don't remember all of them, but I had a much better understanding of what went into building a custom wheelchair by the time we were done.

The second step was to take Jess's measurements: height, weight, the width of her thighs, the length of her shins, torso—you name it, it was measured. After measurements, they started pulling out various chairs to determine what kind of wheels, seat, and back were needed. Who knew that so much went into designing a wheelchair! When they were done, they said it would be about two weeks before the wheelchair was built. They had to send out the order to a custom wheelchair builder since the hospital didn't have all the parts needed for Jess's chair.

So many contraptions were helping Jess get better: the custom wheelchair, the custom helmet protecting her head, the standing machine, the walking machine, the blow-up brace to keep her right leg straight, and even the net bed. In time, Jessica learned to accept the net bed, and I eventually learned to fall asleep to her less frantic marching beat.

We fell into our Holy Cross Hospital routine—Jessica and I. We were inseparable. I was so grateful that I was able to stay with her since everyone else in our family worked full-time jobs, and we were five hours away from home. In the wee hours of every morning, the nurse would slip into the room and place the next day's schedule in the back of the wheelchair. OT, PT, Speech, Cognitive...every waking moment was booked.

Luckily, after lunch, Jess was provided with some downtime for napping. She needed to get a lot of sleep for her brain to heal. I also napped when Jess napped. The exhaustion was threatening to overtake me. I couldn't wait for the weekends to arrive because Jack and Lucy made the five-hour trek right after school on Friday. Emily came along most weekends. I relished the break.

Aaron came on the weekends too. He waited until late Sunday night, though. He always had an excuse for why he couldn't come sooner. His explanations almost always involved Eva's need for his presence in her life— never mind Eva's need for her mother's presence in her life.

Day 25

Leave a Trail

November 20, 2015

Jess's therapy sessions were tiring for her, but she was a trooper. The therapists put her on a machine and "walked" Jessica around the 2nd floor four times. It was very cool to see Jessica upright and looking around as she walked the floor. There is a quote from Ralph Waldo Emerson that hangs on the wall here at Holy Cross Hospital: "Do not go where the path may lead, go instead where there is no path and leave a trail." Jessica was leaving a trail of strength, dignity, love, hope, and faith on this journey, and I was so blessed that I could be a part of the trailblazing.

Chapter 16

UNlovable

The Farm

December 2016

The anger was welling up again. It welled a lot when I was alone with Jessica at Holy Cross Hospital. I found myself pondering all kinds of ways to make Aaron pay for his lack of compassion for his wife and daughter. I'm not sure that's the right word. He lacked compassion, sure, but it was more than that. He lacked empathy. He lacked sympathy. He was just lacking.

I didn't pity him anymore. I didn't concern myself with him other than to express my deep sadness that he refused to bring Eva to see her mother. He didn't care. It was that simple. I guess I kept wishing he would; he was Jessica's husband after all. But as I said before, he wanted to know why this had happened to him.

He appeared to genuinely care when he fought so hard to get Jess transferred to Holy Cross. I wasn't sure why he would fight so hard for his wife one minute and then appear to be completely uncaring the next. The only thing I knew for sure was that public Aaron was utterly different than private Aaron. Public Aaron wanted everyone to see how much he loved his wife. Private Aaron made every excuse in the book to not have to stay with his wife.

To say he was conflicted is an understatement. My feelings toward him were just as conflicted. I wanted to pity him but couldn't. I tried to care about him but couldn't. I wanted to love him, but I simply couldn't do it!

I knew Aaron was still riding high on the pity train at his church. I knew that Aaron and Jessica's friends were still benevolently collecting buckets of cash to help with Jessica's expenses. What I did not know is it wasn't spent on Jessica.

Today is my birthday, but it doesn't mean that I am not feeling the anger or the sadness all over again. I feel both. Feelings are fickle. They don't care if it's your birthday. They show up sometimes and surge to the surface, whether you want them to or not. God. I'm so angry. Hate is an awful word. Hatred is a horrible feeling.

I don't want to name my feelings toward Aaron. I hate what he did to Jessica. I hate what he did to his little family. I hate what he stood for. Do I hate him? Perhaps. It makes me sad to say I hate Aaron because I know my hate doesn't hurt him one bit. It hurts me. It hurts my heart.

My heart is hurting again like it did when I was at Holy Cross Hospital with Jessica. I ignored it for as long as I could. I ignored the tightness in my chest when I was rearranging the furniture in her room. I ignored the squeezing that gripped me the day that Anne, Aaron's mother, showed up and announced that Jessica would come to her house when she left the hospital.

I didn't want to believe that my heart was truly broken—like heart attack broken. Broken, yes. Broken for Jessica. Broken for Eva. Broken for our family, but not broken as in, *I feel like I might have a heart attack.* What kind of broken are we talking about here?

Chapter 17

UNbreakable

Day 26

I have said over and over again that this was a journey of faith. I did believe that God was with us always, but sometimes it helped to be reminded. I felt I was blind sometimes because I could not see the road ahead of me, but isn't that the true meaning of faith? It's believing when you can't see. It's trusting the word of God that the darkness will become light. I had never walked such a walk of faith in my life.

I think that God had been preparing me for this walk for a very long time. I know without a shadow of a doubt that I could not walk this walk without Him. I know that I could not walk this walk without being surrounded by firm believers who lifted Jess and our family in prayer and stood by us through this difficult time. I was and still am grateful for God's word and know that He will keep his promise.

"Thy word is a lamp unto my feet,
And light unto my path" (Ps 119:105 ASV).

Day 27

A Joyful Heart is Good Medicine

November 22, 2015

If laughter is the best medicine, then Emily was a miracle worker. In fact, I believe that she should get her doctorate in laughter because she had Jess laughing up a storm. They started by discussing Jess's one-sided dreadlocks and then went on to laugh at the time Jess's dad took her for a haircut, and she got a mullet. The laughter continued throughout the day, especially when Emily told Jess that her eyebrows were still on point. When they talked about me being on Ambien and the crazy things I did (like chasing the cat around the house naked), they got everyone in the room laughing.

This was the best day yet. Thank goodness for Emily's comic relief. What was even more surprising was that Jess clearly remembered everything and laughed appropriately. This was a huge step in her cognitive development and showed that she was very aware of her surroundings. I didn't want Emily to leave!

Day 29

The New Normal

November 24, 2015

I woke up this morning and thought back to Day 1.

A month ago, Jess's vital systems were shutting down because her brain wasn't communicating with her body. A month ago, Jess's brain activity was minimal at best. A month ago, Jess had a tube draining blood from her brain, and her brain was still swelling. A month ago, Jess had half her skull removed to relieve the swelling. A month ago, we were told she might never breathe on her own.

Last night, Jess went the whole night with her tracheostomy capped (meaning she had to breathe through her mouth and nose), and her oxygen level stayed at 100% the entire night. This indicated that the next step was to remove the tracheostomy and let the hole close on its own (it takes about 72 hours). Today, Jess brushed her own teeth!

So, here's what I'm calling the "new normal" for my daughter, the fighter: The new normal is Jessica walking in the hall with a walking machine. The new normal is Jessica talking and answering questions. The new normal is Jessica brushing her own teeth. The new normal is Jessica taking a spoonful of water and swallowing it. The new normal is Jessica laughing with her sister and kissing everyone who helps her.

This journey was a journey of miracles, and I couldn't help but believe that it was because of the prayers of everyone.

Chapter 18

UNfiltered

Day 39

Jessica "isms"

December 4, 2015

On Day 39, Jessica fired me from taking her out of the wheelchair because I caught my pants on the wheelchair, and Jess ended up on top of me in the bed. As Jess became more and more like herself, her authentic personality was emerging—especially her sense of humor.

Here are just a few of the things Jessica said: She told Emily that she couldn't be a nurse because she didn't have the skills, and she's too careless. Jess said her CNA was her favorite because she "did her dirty work" (changing her diapers). She thanked Aunt Julie for being her special aunt. She asked the PT and OT people if she gave them kisses, would they make her feel better. Then, Jess kissed the lady holding her up. A few minutes later, she told the physical therapist that she didn't think her kisses were working because she wasn't feeling better.

After we sang a bunch of Christmas carols, Jess complained of a headache. Then, she said, "Who wouldn't have a headache after listening to all that noise!" There was a rather handsome doctor that I nicknamed "Dr. Eye Candy." Jess told me Dr. Eye Candy would look good in my workout clothes. She said she has "helmet hair," and the cure for helmet hair is a shower (but she can't take one yet).

She kissed her CNA on the arm and told him that there's more from where that came from. She told Emily that it's really hard to be sneaky around here, especially in the hospital. She told me that she wasn't ready for the family biography, but she did want to say, "Thank you for my wonderful care." I think that about sums it up!

Day 41

Joyful Spirit

December 6, 2015

Jessica arrived at Holy Cross Hospital on November 17th in the "minimally conscious" state. At that time, we were told that she would be there two to three weeks, depending on her level of improvement. She was admitted under the program that specifically focused on "emerging" into the next level of consciousness. If Jessica did not show significant improvement, then she would have gone home after two to three weeks.

However, Jessica showed marked improvement in her cognition and made great strides with her physical limitations as well. Since she showed such improvement, she graduated into the stroke recovery program, which allowed her to stay longer. It was hard to remember the Jessica that came through the doors of Holy Cross Hospital just three weeks before. We knew that she would fight her way back to us, but I think she took us all by surprise with how quickly she progressed.

Her quick wit was an accurate indicator of how intelligent and "with it," she really was. Of course, along with cognition came the reality that things were not the way they used to be. This awakening for Jess was very heart wrenching on so many levels. Sometimes, she just started crying because she was scared. Sometimes, a song would trigger sadness.

Jess was going downstairs for a CAT scan, and we were waiting in the hall. She was scared, so she asked me to sing her a lullaby. I started singing "Puff the Magic Dragon" right there in the hallway. Halfway through the song, Jess began sobbing. I asked her what was wrong, and she said, "Please don't sing songs that make me sad." "Puff the Magic Dragon" is the song that she never remembers all the words to, so she and I sing it together to Eva. I know she was thinking of Eva, and it broke my heart in a million pieces. I know those periods of sadness were as necessary as the periods of laughter, but I found it so hard to see her feeling so sad. I felt totally helpless.

Thankfully, those periods were not as frequent as the times of laughter and fun. Jessica had such a joyful spirit that just kept shining through. She said that she was Mike Tyson with her boxing glove on (the soft-cushioned glove that kept her from hurting herself when she marched in place), but she hadn't bitten anyone's ear off yet. Although, she did threaten to bite the OT therapist if he didn't stop moving her left arm (she was just kidding, of course).

I couldn't help but think that this verse summed up what it would be like when Jessica fully emerged: "For ye shall go out with joy, and be led forth with peace: the mountains and the hills shall break forth before you into singing; and all the trees of the fields shall clap their hands" (Isaiah 55:12).

Day 48

The Wall of Inspiration

December 13, 2015

As the days passed, Jess and I began having more and more in-depth conversations. She was very blunt and asked pointed questions. For instance, she wanted to know if Jack and I were going to stay married because I didn't kiss him enough. She made me list all the things I loved about her dad to reassure her that I still loved him. It had been a long time since I thought about all the things I loved about her dad. I think it should be a requirement for all married couples since we tend to forget how important we are to each other and why.

Jess was well aware of the care she was receiving and never failed to thank everyone involved in her care. Although I'd been fired on numerous occasions, from getting her out of the wheelchair to feeding her, she never failed to thank me for taking such good care of her. When the man screaming across the hall woke her at night, she didn't say, "I wish he'd shut up!" No, she asked me to check on him, and we prayed for him over and over again.

She was becoming aware of her progress, too, and worried that she was not making enough headway. We spent a lot of time going to the Wall of Inspiration. We would read all the inspiring stories of people who had been at Holy Cross Hospital and now worked here or had accomplished great goals. Her goal was to make it on the wall of inspiration. I had no doubt she would.

I thought that it would be a great idea to create a wall of inspiration in Jess's home. Perhaps we should all have walls of inspiration. On Jess's wall of inspiration, I would list this week's considerable accomplishments. Jess fed herself, she straightened her left leg on her own, she stood for a minute in the standing machine without anyone helping her find her center of balance, and she sat on her own (balancing for a minute without any assistance).

Jess walked through the hall in the walking machine, bending and straightening her left leg on her own. She wrote out a grocery list on a whiteboard, she unscrambled five-word sentences, she made nine baskets playing basketball—all the while asking, "Am I making progress?" Jessica was my inspiration! She was my hero. I was so proud and humbled to call her my daughter.

Day 52

Hope for the Future

December 17, 2015

I was sitting by the window next to Jess's bed, and the light was shining through in such a way that it highlighted her green eyes when she looked at me. I looked into her eyes, and I felt as though I were looking into her soul. I saw a depth of sadness in her eyes that I hadn't seen before. This was a sad day for Jess. She was missing Eva so very much. Aaron had left to go home, and I knew it was very hard on the family. I just wanted to take the sadness away from her, but I knew it was as necessary for her healing as it was for her to experience joy.

It was so hard not finding the words to comfort her. It was hard when my *own* sadness threatened to well up and pour out like a rushing river. I knew, as hard as it was, I had to let Jessica see all the emotions that accompany our journey. She needed to know that it was okay and necessary for her to be able to express her sadness and her fears. I needed to express those emotions, as well.

We were entering a difficult time because reality was creeping up on all of us. The awareness of medical bills and lost income weighed heavily on Aaron. The

135

reality of how different home was going to be was especially hard for Jessica. The fear of the unknown was a constant companion for all of us. I had to continually remind myself and Jessica how far she had come from where she had been two months before. When we looked back on where she had been, the future looked so much brighter.

I took Jess to have an ultrasound. The technician was the same technician that did her ultrasound shortly after Jess arrived. At that time, the technician said that Jessica was only blowing kisses. She couldn't believe all the progress Jess had made since then. Everyone was amazed at Jess's tenacity and drive to get well. She was exceeding all expectations, as we all knew she would. Her discharge date had been extended to January 14th, which meant that she continued to make great strides, and they believed they could prove to the insurance company that she would continue to make marked improvements.

A week before, Jess was sitting for 30 seconds on her own. Today, Jess sat for 30 minutes on her own and was very close to standing by herself! She was reading things that were on her left side, something she could not do the previous week. Jess was starting to regain feeling in her left arm and leg as well. Every day brought new milestones and new emotions. Jessica was still so positive, yet she knew that things would be very different, and I knew that sometimes those worries started to overwhelm her.

Reflection

It is common for brain aneurysm survivors to become overwhelmed. This phenomenon is often referred to as "flooding" because the individual is flooded with all kinds of emotions at once, and the brain injury makes it difficult, if not impossible, to sort out the inundation of feelings.

Day 57

Christmas Miracle

December 22, 2015

We all think of Christmas as a time of great joy and happiness. It's a time to celebrate the birth of our savior and spend time with family and friends. The joyful Christmas story is full of drama and struggles too. I can't imagine how Mary must have felt riding a donkey while being nine months pregnant and then giving birth in a stable. I don't even want to think about the trials Joseph endured trying to make his wife as comfortable as possible, given the obstacles they were facing. Yet, they endured, and they triumphed in a stable surrounded by sheep and cattle.

The birth of our savior is a very human story, isn't it? It tells of the fortitude and tenacity of the human spirit. Everyone loves a great human spirit story. It gives us hope. It makes us look at our own lives and take stock in what matters most. Jessica's journey is such a story.

This journey was not without its drama. Our family had its share of struggles over the first two months. We wouldn't be human if we didn't disagree and argue, but we always found our way back to one another. We continually reminded each other that Jessica was our priority, and she deserved our cooperation.

I learned a lot about myself and my family. I learned who was patient and who was hot-headed. I learned who the peacemakers were and who the warriors were. I learned that we needed both the warriors and the peacemakers because each played an essential role in this journey. I learned that, despite the differences, we had a family that loved deeply and had an unwavering faith that God would see us through. Like the Christmas story, we had endured so many obstacles. Together we faced them, and together we would triumph. We all knew that the Christmas story doesn't end with the birth of Jesus in a manger. It was just the beginning.

I knew in my heart that Jess's story was just the beginning of a miraculous journey for her and our family. I knew that her journey had already touched so many, and I believed that it would continue to do so. Jessica was our Christmas miracle. She was living proof of God's mighty healing powers. I cannot even imagine what God had in store for her. I just knew that whatever came Jess's way, she would face everything with strength and dignity, and she would laugh at the days to come (especially at her dysfunctional family).

Day 60

Merry Christmas from Jess

December 25, 2015

As a Christmas gift to all our Caring Bridge readers, Jess wanted to share some thoughts. She did the talking, and I did the typing. Jess's words:

> First of all, I want to wish everyone a Merry Christmas. I'm sorry that everyone missed my family's singing Christmas carols. Actually, I'm glad everyone missed my family singing! Today we played Family Feud, and I was the team captain. Our team won. Christmas is a special time to spend with friends and family, and I wish I could spend it with everyone who reads Caring Bridge. I love all of you. Sweet dreams.
> Love, Jess

Day 63

A Birthday Wish

December 28, 2015

The day before my birthday, Jessica asked me what I wanted for my birthday. At that moment, I told her that I had everything I need: my entire family all healthy (or getting healthier) and a place to call home. This caused me to reflect on the many birthday gifts I'd received in the past. Of course, the ones that meant the most to me were always the gifts from the heart.

My son Kevin gave me a gift one time, which was a picture that I drew for him when he first came to live with us as a foster child. The picture had obviously been folded and battered over the more than 20 years since I had drawn the stick figure family. The drawing included Kevin and his brother in the front yard playing a game of some sort. There was a peculiar looking cat on the roof of the house that was way too big in proportion to the rest of the picture.

Kevin said it was because he loved the cat, so I drew it bigger. In any case, the picture looked as if a five-year-old drew it—a testament to my drawing abilities. What surprised me is that Kevin clearly treasured that picture enough to keep it for over 20 years and then frame it and give it to me on my birthday.

The picture was accompanied by a letter telling me how much it meant to Kevin to have a place to call home where he and his brother were loved and wanted. Isn't that what we all long for in our hearts? Isn't that what pulls at our heartstrings when we see homeless people? We wonder what it would be like not to have people around you who love you and make you feel safe.

I was so thankful that Jessica was surrounded by people who loved her and made her feel safe. My birthday wish was that she continue to feel loved and safe, especially as she began to make her transition to home. Jessica continued to make great strides every day. Her cognition and ability to understand what happened to her were getting clearer for her. With that clarity came some fears and frustration, especially about her short-term memory.

I knew that going home weighed heavily on her mind because she worried about how she would handle the future. Of course, I had every confidence that she would handle the future with the same tenacity and grace that had taken her this far in her recovery.

So, as Jessica moved closer to leaving Holy Cross Hospital, my prayer for her and her family was that all of them would know the comfort of a place to call home where they could all feel secure and loved.

I was so blessed to have a husband and children that sacrificed so much to give me the freedom to be here with Jessica as she recovered and who kept the home fires burning in my absence. I was so blessed to have extended family and friends that helped in many ways. I couldn't have asked for a better birthday present than the immeasurable support we received from everyone.

Day 65

Trust

December 30, 2015

As we transitioned into the New Year, it was hard to believe how far Jess had come since the first day when she wasn't talking or able to breathe without help. Every time I left, even for a short time, I returned to learn of some new milestone. Jess still could not walk on her own, but she was able to move both her legs with help and made it around the nurse's station in just over three minutes using the walking machine.

The walking machine required two people moving Jess's legs and feet with one person in front and one behind Jess to help her balance. When she first started walking in the machine, it was taking over 12 minutes to make it once around the floor.

Jess wasn't able to sit on her own when she arrived, and now she could sit without assistance. Standing was getting much better. She was able to balance and hold it for over a minute (with some help). Jess was able to stand and press buttons that lit up to her left. This was very impressive because Jess was unable to look to her left when she first arrived.

She suffered from "left neglect," which is common for someone who has a right-brain stroke. Left neglect essentially means that the patient forgets they have a left side. It is challenging to overcome left neglect because the brain has to be retrained to acknowledge the affected side.

This requires constant training, which is extremely tiring for the patient. Jess's training consisted of wearing specialized glasses that limited the vision on her right side while encouraging her to use her left eye. She also had to reach across her body with her right arm and do activities on her left side. This was extremely difficult for Jess, but she persisted.

Then, she beat a record of 17 buttons. While standing for one minute, she pressed 28 buttons on her left side! That's not all Mighty Mouse (her new nickname) did. She had to read directions and write the answers on the lines to her left. For instance, she had to read the direction: Write the name of a person next to number 3 in the left column. Not only did she read the instructions, but she also followed the directions without assistance. I was honored that she wrote my name.

The writing activity had ten instructions requiring her to write the answers in both the left and right columns. She performed the entire exercise in 15 minutes. Two days before, Jess was unable to complete this task. Still, Jess said she didn't feel like she was making progress. I consistently reminded her how far she had come.

It was so sweet when we were in the hall with a young lady who was waiting for OT. The young lady just had her trach capped and was trying to talk to her mother. Jess looked over at her and said, "Don't worry, the therapists tell me it gets better every day, and I trust them."

It was hard to believe that just a month before, Jess could only communicate with kisses, and now she was encouraging her peers in her own words.

Chapter 19

UNagreeable

"Discharge Plans"

January 2016

As Jess's discharge date grew closer, I became more and more concerned about her future. Thus far, I had been the primary caregiver for Jess with very little help from Aaron. He was not at all hands-on with Jess even when he came for his weekend visits. I worried that he wouldn't be able to handle the day in and day out responsibilities that would accompany her homecoming. This weighed heavily on my mind, and I expressed these concerns to the social worker at Holy Cross.

She was supposed to be holding Aaron accountable for presenting a discharge plan to Jess's team of doctors, nurses, therapists, and psychologists. To add to my apprehension, I was not consulted about what my role would be after Jess's discharge. I learned that there was a "caring for Jess" meeting scheduled with Anne, Aaron's mom, who had only been to the hospital twice since Jess arrived at Holy Cross. Anne's two visits were short and sweet, with little interaction between Jess and her mother-in-law.

I witnessed a few conversations that mostly centered on Eva since Anne was the primary caregiver of Eva while Aaron was at work. I did not observe Anne transferring Jess from her wheelchair to bed or the toilet. Anne did not assist with bathing Jess or helping with her therapy sessions. Mostly, Anne's visits consisted of sitting in Jess's room and keeping her company for short periods.

So, I was surprised that Anne would be attending a meeting about caring for Jess. It was evident that she didn't want to take on that responsibility during her infrequent hospital visits, which were followed by a rapid departure. Come to think of it, Anne was non-existent when we needed volunteers to stay with Jess overnight at Memorial Hospital.

The caring for Jess meeting took place on a Saturday. Aaron wasn't present.

Before the meeting even began, Anne (flanked by her significant other, Steve), came into Jess's room and announced to Jess that she was so excited that Jess would be coming to live with them. I couldn't believe my ears. I kept my mouth shut, though, for Jess's sake, and figured we'd hash everything out in the caring for Jess meeting.

Steve seemed like a nice enough guy. He was always pleasant and usually smiling. I just couldn't picture Jess being alone with Steve while Anne and Aaron were at work. I wasn't comfortable with this idea at all!

My sister and I nicknamed Steve, Sponge Steve. We named him Sponge Steve because he was sort of shaped like Sponge Bob, and he resembled a sponge in other ways. Sponge Steve was smiling ear to ear as Anne announced Jess would be moving in with them. I wasn't sure what was making him so happy. I honestly didn't know what to think.

Jess didn't say anything to either of them. She just looked confused. I said it would be best if we all discussed this with the social worker at the discharge meeting. Then, I left the room before I said something I'd regret. I didn't want to add any stress to Jess.

The discharge meeting soon followed, but neither Jess nor I were informed of the meeting. I just happened to learn of it from Jess's nurse when I came back into Jess's room after I had made a trip to the hotel to take a shower. The nurse told me I'd better hoof it to the social worker's office if I wanted to have any input in the discharge plans. I quickly made my way to the social worker's hallway.

Sponge Steve and Anne began speaking to me as soon as I opened the door to the office where Jess's discharge meeting was taking place—minus Jess, of course.

"I just want you to know," said Sponge Steve with a hint of callousness in his voice, "we want to give you a break for a while. You've carried your share of the load so far. Our family will take care of Jess now. You'll be able to visit her, of course, but you'll just have to call first. We don't want the house to become a circus with people coming in and out constantly."

Anne sat stoically on her metal chair, her jowls drooping bulldog-like. "We appreciate all you've done for Jess, and it is our turn now."

I could have responded with a spirit of thankfulness, but I didn't. I wasn't feeling thankful at that moment. I was feeling ambushed since they hadn't given me any information about the discharge plan. I didn't know that Jess's side of the family (parents, siblings, aunts, uncles, and extended family) was going to play second fiddle, even though only Jess's side of the family had been intimately involved with her daily care.

"You've got to be kidding me!" I yelled at the two of them as I took a seat in the cramped office of Darlene Shire—social worker extraordinaire. At that moment, I felt like wiping Darlene's smug smile right off her face.

"What the hell are you talking about?" I screamed. "Why wouldn't Jess's family continue to be part of her care? I thought we were meeting to discuss Jessica's discharge plan for all of us, Jessica's family as well as yours." I glared at Darlene. "Where the hell is Jessica? Doesn't she have a say in this?"

Darlene tried to calm me down. "I don't think you need to be in this meeting since you've been here at the hospital the entire time, and you know how to take care of Jessica," she soothed through her fake smile. "Aaron told me that Jessica is fine with living at Anne's, so we don't really need to include Jess in this meeting either. You can leave if you want," she said, dismissively turning her back to me so she could face the sponge and bulldog. "You might want to give Jessica a basket to carry the remote...."

"A basket for the remote!" my shouting interrupted her. "What the fuck are you talking about?"

I don't usually curse. I'm not proud of my word choice. I could have left this out of the book, but the story would not be real if I did. It takes a lot for me to throw the "F" bomb, but, at that moment, I was letting my temper get the best of me, and I dropped that word like it was a hand grenade. The irrelevance of a basket for the remote was just too absurd for me not to react. In the scheme of things, there were far more pressing issues Darlene needed to address.

Darlene was not discussing how to toilet Jess. She wasn't reviewing the series of daily exercises or telling them how to help Jess with eating or her cognitive development. I expected this meeting to include Jessica's team of therapists as well as her doctors. Darlene was not at the top of my list of qualified people caring for Jess. In fact, she didn't even make the list.

I came to all of Darlene's group sessions with Jess. Within the month, Jess was practically running the group. Like the teacher she was, Jess asked all the new people to point to the calendar and clock before Darlene could even begin the group. It was comical to a degree because it was clear that Darlene was happy to have Jess running her class—less work for her.

Sometimes there are just certain words that satisfy like none other. Perhaps it was the dropping of the "F" bomb that earned me the nickname of "Drama Momma," as Sponge Steve posted on Facebook shortly after our discharge meeting. He's such a witty guy.

Facebook can get you into trouble quickly. This is especially true for hotheaded people like me and Sponge Steve. My Facebook faux pas consisted of me asking Aaron if Eva possessed a "mommy tee shirt" after he posted a picture of Eva in her "daddy tee shirt" at bedtime. Apparently, I was causing drama by asking such a provocative question. It didn't matter that there was not a single picture or mention of Jess on Aaron's Facebook page for months.

Sponge Steve went after me like a dog with a bone. Hence, I earned the title of Drama Momma courtesy of Steve. I like it. It suits me. I'm happy to report that I didn't stoop to his level and call him Sponge Steve on Facebook, and I even deleted the thread.

Speaking of thread—my yarn is spinning too fast. I'm not done telling the story of the discharge meeting.

So, I was saying that I had everyone's attention. I knew because they were all staring blankly at me, perhaps waiting for the next "F" bomb. I proceeded to yell. My focus was on Darlene now.

"These two have not spent so much as one day with Jessica in the past three months!" I spat, pointing at Bulldog Anne and Sponge Steve. "How are they supposed to know what she needs? Are any of you aware of the fact that Jessica has said over and over that she wishes to return to her *own* home with her daughter and husband?"

"She doesn't want to live with you, Anne. She has made that abundantly clear to her nurses and me. Have any of you consulted her nurses? Aaron is not here enough to know what Jessica wants. He tells her what *he* wants and then tells everyone that Jess agrees with him. He doesn't listen to her. Right now, no one at this hospital is listening to her!"

I stood, and I'm sure my face was turning as crimson as the burning rage inside of me. It felt like an invisible hand reached into my chest and took a firm grasp of my heart then, and I found it hard to breathe. I made a hasty exit before anyone realized my heart was about to explode.

"I've had enough of this bullshit!" I shouted as the door slammed in my wake. I walked down the hall to Jess's room, feeling battered and bruised as if I had just gone several rounds in a prizefight. I may have been down for the count, but I was not giving up this fight. How dare they tell me that they'll be caring for Jess now and that I'd have to call before I came over.

I opened the door to Jess's room to find my sister-in-law Julie reading a book while Jess napped. This was Julie's week to help care for Jessica. Julie and my sister Lisa alternated weeks so I could get some rest. No one from Aaron's extended family had come to stay—ever. We were at Holy Cross Hospital from November through February, ample time for someone from his family to make an effort to learn how to care for Jess.

Bulldog Anne and Ostrich Aunt came once with Aaron, but they only stayed for about an hour and went to the hotel afterward. I remember that day well. Jack was there, so it had to be a weekend day, one of the few weekend days that Aaron came early (probably because his mother and aunt were with him). I was so looking forward to going to the hotel that night with my husband. Both Jack and I assumed that Aaron would stay at the hospital with his wife. We were wrong.

When Mommy Dearest and Ostrich Aunt announced they were going to the hotel, Aaron got up and started to leave with them. Jack stopped him.

"Where are you going, Aaron?" Jack asked.

"To the hotel. I have to drive them there. They don't know where it is," Aaron said defensively as he pointed to his mom and aunt.

"They can drive your truck and follow us," Jack said. "Gwen needs to rest. We're going back to the hotel."

Mommy and aunty quickly interrupted Jack.

"You don't expect him to try to sleep on that couch and then drive five hours tomorrow, do you?" Anne's righteous indignation dripped from her voice.

"Aaron needs his rest," Ostrich Aunt interjected. "Gwen isn't driving anywhere tomorrow. She can sleep tomorrow."

My heart was bleeding for poor baby Aaron who was exhausted from making the five-hour trip after working all day. I couldn't stand to listen to this exchange any longer and in front of Jessica no less. What the hell did they think? Did they think that Jess was a vegetable unable to hear the heated exchange over who would be burdened with staying the night with her?

I stormed out of the room and made my way to the recreation room, where I could be alone with my thoughts. Jack found me after about an hour, and he told me that Aaron would be staying the night with Jess. I didn't ask what transpired after my departure, but I surmised that Jack was influential in the decision making. Thankfully, we were going back to the hotel. Jack told me that the mother and aunt had already left and would use the GPS to get them safely to the hotel.

Chapter 20

UNbearable

Holy Cross Hospital

January 2016

Holy Cross Hospital was a true blessing for Jess. Even though Jess celebrated Thanksgiving and Christmas at the hospital, they made sure that she and her family were provided with the opportunity to make both holidays as enjoyable as possible in a hospital setting. Jess spent both holidays with Jack and me, her aunts, uncles, siblings, and even one of my closest friends, "Grandma Carol," and her son Bill.

Aaron didn't come. He celebrated both holidays at his mother's house. Eva too. Eva didn't see her mommy on Thanksgiving or Christmas. Mommy, Eva was told by Aaron, was still getting her boo-boo fixed by the doctors.

I can recall yelling furiously at Aaron on more than one occasion. "I'll tell you one thing, Aaron. If I were Eva, I'd be scared shitless if I got a boo-boo!"

By the time the infamous "discharge meeting" with Aaron's mom, Sponge Steve, and I came around, Aaron and I had already had our share of knock-down, drag-out fights over Eva seeing her mommy.

Anne and I also had a texting battle on Christmas day. Anne accused me of ruining Aaron's day because Jack told Aaron that Jessica woke up that morning crying for her daughter and continued to cry for about two hours. I don't know how that equated to me ruining

Aaron's day, but somehow, I got blamed for everything. I didn't care, though. I wanted Aaron's day to be ruined.

Here is Anne's text to me:

> Do you think you could have made this day any worse for Aaron? You need to respect his decisions. Jess doesn't remember FaceTime. So, if he brought Eva, she wouldn't remember the next day, but Eva would. That means taking our granddaughter away from her mommy and hurting her. He won't allow that. You need to back off. She added, Jess has and always will be Eva's mommy.

It figures that Anne would talk about how Aaron's day was ruined—nothing about Jessica's day or Eva's day. Oh well, I guess that is why Anne raised the kind of boy Aaron became. It's probably the reason Aaron has never reached manhood. I imagine it's why Aaron hired the "Men's Rights Law Firm" to represent him in the divorce because all sniveling momma's boys hire men's rights law firms.

My text to Anne was simple and to the point. I told her that it was Jack who contacted Aaron while I was busy trying to cook a ham in a crockpot in the hotel room. I explained that I've already told Aaron how I feel about Eva seeing her mother—especially on Christmas day. I wanted to say so much more. I did write her a letter that I never sent. Writing helps me deal with my anger without actually saying something I would regret later. Here's my letter that I guess I held onto for posterity's sake:

Anne,

You asked me if I could have made this day any worse for Aaron. Aaron decided to NOT spend the day with his wife and daughter. I didn't make that choice—he did. We had to deal with the fallout from his decision with our sobbing, inconsolable daughter who wanted to be with her daughter. I could ask you the same question: Could Aaron have made this day any worse for Jess? If Aaron is smart enough to handle Eva's missing her mom with such finesse and skill, I have no doubt he could handle Eva seeing her mother with that same finesse and skill.

Meanwhile, his wife, my daughter, your daughter-in-law, and Eva's mother cries every day and longs in her heart to see and touch her child. Yes, I could have made the day worse for Aaron. I could have put him on the phone and told him to console his wife. I could have told *him* to explain why Jess can't see Eva, but I didn't, to protect Jess. Instead, we consoled her as best we could, and we tried to make the day as pleasant as possible.

Jessica knows full well who is keeping Eva from her, and as I told you before, I believe he'll pay a dear price for his decision. You told me to back off, Anne. Let me make one thing perfectly clear to you: When it comes to protecting my daughter and her daughter, I will NEVER back off!

Anger smoldering, my temper was still flaring when I stomped into Jess's room after the discharge meeting. Jess's Aunt Julie looked up at me expectantly as I entered the room.

"That went well," I informed Julie. "I'm not feeling so great. I think I'll go back to the hotel and take a nap if it's okay with you. I'll fill you in on the meeting after my nap."

That night, out of earshot of Jess, I filled Julie in on all the details of the discharge meeting. With every utterance of Anne's and Steve's names, I felt my blood pressure rise. I cried and carried on like a blubbering fool while Julie added fuel to my fire with words like: "Those bastards!"

Anger is like that; it rears its ugly head every time you feed it. My fury wanted to be fed often, and well. I took great care of my anger. I let it rage inside of me like a runaway virus—even to the point where it infected every pore. It poisoned my soul, and it overwhelmed my heart.

The next day, I asked Julie if she would stay with Jessica for a few days because I probably should go home and get my heart checked; it was hurting a little. Anne and Sponge Steve had already made their hurried departure after the discharge meeting, although they were supposed to stay one more night and come back to the hospital the next day for training with her therapists and doctors on how to care for Jess. Evidently, Steve's diabetes was acting up, and his foot was hurting him, so they had to leave.

I had to wonder how they would be able to care for Jess if Sponge Steve was hindered by his foot, and Bulldog Anne had to work. Who would be home with Jess? Who knew how to lift and move Jess? Neither of them knew what Jess was working on to improve her cognition. They didn't know how to shower or dress her. They didn't know how to help her brush her teeth. They didn't know her exercise routine. Surely, they didn't expect Sponge Steve to take Jess to the bathroom.

I know that Jess had told Aaron she didn't want Steve taking her to the bathroom or helping her shower. Poor Jess, I can't imagine how completely helpless and afraid she felt about her future. Jess had no control at all over the decisions Aaron was making for her—not with her. My heart ached for my daughter.

Day 69

Countdown

January 3, 2016

Jessica was in countdown mode. She had been asking everyone who came into her room if they could get her out of there. Every morning before she even got out of bed, we got the calendar out and counted the days until she would go home. Each day Jess crossed off was one day closer to being with Eva and Aaron. Right now, that was her motivation for continuing to work hard. It broke my heart to know how much Jessica longed to hold her baby.

Jess worried about not being able to hold Eva in both her arms (her left arm was still paralyzed). She worried that she could not be the mother that she was to Eva. I knew in my heart that Jess was an amazing mother and would continue to be an amazing mother to her beautiful daughter. I also knew that Eva was looking forward to being a big helper for Mommy. Their reunion would be a day of immeasurable joy. Until that day, Jess knew that therapy must continue.

Little by little, the staff was turning over the reins to me so I could learn the proper techniques for moving Jess by myself and helping her get through her day. Jessica was able to help more and more each day. She was able to stand while I held her and moved her to her wheelchair. She helped me when I had to reposition her in bed to get her dressed or sit her up.

There are so many things we take for granted every day (like brushing our teeth) that I had to learn to assist Jess with. While showering Jess, I managed to give myself and the CNA a shower as well. Jessica worried that going home would present a whole new set of challenges without the Holy Cross Hospital staff there to help. Every day, I had to reassure her that her family would all be there to help her, and she wouldn't have to fire us for doing a terrible job (even though I still got fired almost every day).

Jessica was scheduled to return home on January 14th. So, the following two weeks would be spent preparing her and the family for her homecoming. The journey to healing and becoming whole was far from over for Jess. This was just a new chapter in her remarkable story.

Day 72

Another Bump in the Road
Written by Jack

January 6, 2016

As most of you know, Gwen has been up in Jacksonville with Jess since her arrival there seven weeks ago. It's been a remarkable journey, but it has taken its toll on all of us, especially Gwen, who has done the vast majority of caretaking. Last Saturday, I got a call from Gwen telling me that she has had chest pains, shortness of breath, and numbness in her left arm for the past two weeks. She was hoping it would go away because she really wanted to finish out this journey in Jacksonville with Jess until January 14th (her discharge date). Even the few times Gwen has come back home, her heart and spirit were up in Jacksonville, and she couldn't wait to get back to Jess.

I drove up to Jacksonville to get her the next day after her phone call and brought her back home. She went to see her cardiologist and went through several different stress tests. Today she was told to get over to the hospital immediately because there was a major blockage in her heart. She was taken into emergency surgery and had two stents placed in her left anterior descending artery (LAD). That artery had a 95%

blockage (often known as the widowmaker because it usually happens to men and is almost always fatal). On Friday, she will have three stents put in her right coronary artery (RCA).

She is resting and recuperating at the hospital and will hopefully be home soon. Please keep her in your thoughts and prayers. I do not doubt that she will bounce back and play an important role in Jessica's recovery once she gets home. Jess does not know about this situation, and we would prefer she wasn't told at this point. She is stressing out enough about her extended stay and getting back to her family.

Day 74

I Don't Get It!
Written by Jack

January 8, 2016

The last two and a half months have been a mystery to me. I've seen my very healthy 29-year-old daughter collapse during a morning run and end up with a brain aneurysm and stroke. Despite all odds, she has bounced back and made remarkable progress. Believe me, she has a long way to go, but with her courage and strength, there is no doubt in my mind she will make it back.

My question with Jess is, how do you take the nicest, sweetest person I know and put her through this? I don't get it. Added to this mystery is the recent tragedy of my wife, Gwen, who has been by Jess's side throughout this whole journey. As most of you know, Gwen had to come home last weekend because of health concerns.

Thank God she did because the doctor who put in the stents said she was fortunate to be alive. Yesterday she got an intense headache and started throwing up, which resulted in her getting a CAT scan. Unfortunately, the CAT scan revealed bleeding to the back of her brain. They believe the bleeding has stopped, and we are now in the waiting process. If the swelling gets worse, they will have to go in and relieve the bleeding. Hopefully, it won't, and the body will absorb the blood, and she'll be fine.

I know that all of these recent events have taken a toll on the whole family. I can only hope that having Jessica home with us soon will relieve some of these worries and stress that we are all feeling. Especially for Gwen, who wants more than anything to be by Jessica's side through this time as she has been her entire stay at Holy Cross Hospital. I know Jess and Eva finally being reunited will mean the world to both of them. A big key in Jessica's progress is that we all unite as a team and work together in her best interest.

I have a big concern about this because at the discharge meeting this afternoon that Emily and I attended, with Aaron on speakerphone, it was revealed that none of the members of Jess's family were even included on the care-taker team. Aaron told us that we could visit Jess as long as we phoned ahead. It seems that the doctors and other team members at Holy Cross Hospital did not object to the plan. Once again, I don't get it. Please keep your prayers and positive thoughts coming. We will truly need them as we move on through this journey.

Chapter 21

UNwrapped

The Farm

December 2016

By January, Jessica had made tremendous progress. Although she was still missing half her skull from the surgery, she had been weaned off the tracheostomy tube, had the feeding tube removed, was talking, and was no longer perpetually marching in place.

Dr. Eye Candy was the doctor who performed the minor procedure of removing the tracheostomy tube. He asked me to assist him since it was a weekend, and there was a skeleton nursing staff on the floor.

"Can you just help me by handing me the items I need to close the hole?" he asked pleasantly.

My eyes were fixated on Dr. Eye Candy's baby blue eyes and toned arms, so his words sort of floated by me without really registering.

"Sure," I said dreamily.

"Please wash your hands," he said. "Put on the gloves that are on the tray and join me over here."

"Ok," I responded as I made my way to the bathroom to wash my hands for surgery. I put the gloves on like a pro—snapping the fingers as they do on TV.

I stood right next to Dr. Eye Candy with my eyes fixated on Jess as he bent over Jess and told her that he was going to remove the tube in her neck because she no longer needed it. I was so proud of myself because I never took my eyes off of Jess as Dr. Eye Candy bent over—not once.

Jess looked a little scared, but she's a trooper and didn't flinch or look like she was going to try and bolt from the bed. However, her expression turned to fear when Dr. Eye Candy said, "Your mom is going to assist me."

Perhaps Jess understood that my attention might be diverted from the surgery by Dr. Eye Candy's muscles, but I hoped that she'd give me more credit than that.

Anyway, Dr. Eye Candy started by cleaning around the tracheostomy, and then he began pulling on the tube. At first, I was a bit fascinated by the procedure. Soon, I became a tad nauseous as the mucus-covered tube just kept getting longer and longer. When it was finally out, I could see right into Jess's windpipe through the hole in her neck. I wanted to puke at this point, but that wouldn't be very ladylike, so I remained by Dr. Eye Candy's side like the adept surgical assistant I had become.

I stifled my urge to say, "What do you need, Doctor?"

"Will you please hand me the gauze?" Dr. Eye Candy reached out his hand towards me.

Gauze, I thought, *where's the gauze? I can't find the gauze!*

Dr. Eye Candy pointed to the tray behind me as he held his gloved hand over the hole in Jess's neck.

I grabbed the box of gauze and placed it neatly in Dr. Eye Candy's hand.

"Can you take one out and unwrap it?" he asked, still holding his hand over the hole in Jess's neck.

"Oops," I said, laughing.

Dr. Eye Candy didn't laugh.

"Please hand me the numbing spray." He reached out his hand. I put the numbing spray in his hand with great finesse. Next, he asked me to hand him the suture thingy that was already threaded.

I held it up so I wouldn't stab him.

This is easy, I thought. Then, Dr. Eye Candy asked me to hold the hole closed while he stitched it together.

"What?" I said with a hint of trepidation.

"All you have to do is come to the other side of the bed and pinch these two pieces of skin together while I sew the hole closed," he coaxed. "It's not difficult."

Jess was looking a bit wide-eyed at this point, and I didn't want her to sense my dismay, so I walked to the other side of the bed, reached over to the hole and pinched the skin together, all the while praying that I wouldn't faint. I didn't faint, and the sewing only took about a minute.

After the procedure, Dr. Eye Candy told me I could assist him at any time. I'm not sure, but I think this remark might have been a bit sarcastic.

After he left, Jess fired me from being Dr. Eye Candy's assistant because my attention was not on the task at hand. I started to protest, but the truth is that Dr. Eye Candy's physique may have been a bit distracting during surgery.

Jessica, the butterfly, had emerged from her cocoon and was spreading her wings. Not flying yet—not even walking—but she was well on her way to understanding a lot about what happened to her. Of course, she was still in the wheelchair, still required assistance in the bathroom, and still had to wear a helmet to protect her head, but her overall improvement was nothing short of a miracle.

Jessica was still in need of lots of physical assistance with activities of daily living, and I was terrified that Aaron, Bulldog Anne, Ostrich Aunt, and Sponge Steve would be her only lifeline once she left Holy Cross Hospital.

I didn't despise Anne, yet. I disliked her immensely because she coddled Aaron and never stood up to him about Eva. I knew that Anne was perfectly happy with the current arrangement because she got the prize—Eva. Eva was with Anne in her home, and Anne had complete control over who could see her and when. My gut told me that Aaron's family had already diminished Jessica in Eva's eyes and that Jessica would play little if any, role in her daughter's life when she went to live with Anne.

Diminishing a mother is something I was all too familiar with, so, understandably, I would fight to the nth degree to keep Jessica's mommy role in Eva's life. I tried. God knows I tried. Thinking back to Anne's particularly awful text, I remember Anne's words: "Jessica was and will always be Eva's mommy." Really? Not in Anne's household. I knew this without a shadow of a doubt. I knew it in my gut, and there was very little I could do about it.

Even though Eva hadn't seen Jessica and had barely spoken with her mother on the phone for three months, Anne had the nerve to think that I would believe her "always will be her mommy" text. The fact that Aaron was refusing to budge on any interaction between Jess and Eva seemed to be just fine with Anne.

She protected her son and defended his actions at all costs. It was fine with Anne that Eva didn't attend the prayer vigil for her mom. Anne helped Aaron perpetuate the boo-boo myth.

What's wrong with telling Eva over and over that the doctors were still fixing her mommy's boo-boo? *Everyone* goes away for months to get a boo-boo fixed. Mommy went to get her boo-boo fixed. Mommy went to the store. What does it matter what you tell a child? Mommy is still gone!

No, I didn't despise Anne at first. I learned to detest her as time went on, and she continued to allow Aaron to perfect his victim role without so much as an "I told you so." No reprimand.

I continued my push for Jess and Eva's relationship restoration, but the truth is, I was sick—very sick. I was also exhausted. I fought a hard battle that I may have lost, but I still thought I'd win the war over Eva. I'd win the war because I would never give up. I'd win the war because I was older and wiser than Aaron. I'd win the war because I knew what was at stake. In Aaron's brain, this was just a battle for control. He could not comprehend the damage he was inflicting on his child, but I knew firsthand what it was like to be lied to by the adults in your life that were entrusted to protect you.

I can't ever forget the little girl that was me. I can't ever forget how much I missed my mommy, who did go away and never came back. I was never told the truth. I had to learn about my mother's death when I was old enough to ask the right questions and request the autopsy on my own. I waited for 20 years to learn that my mother died after suffering a heart attack and other complications. I believe that God allowed the pain of losing my mother in my life so that I could fight the good fight for Jess and Eva.

I went to live with my aunt and remembered nothing about my mom. The emotions are still there, though. The scars haven't healed completely. They fester and ooze with sadness from time to time, like when I looked at Jess in the hospital and noticed the faraway daze in her eyes, and I knew that she was thinking about Eva. The wounds oozed and bled for my granddaughter, who I knew was missing her mommy.

I wanted so much to tell Eva the truth. I felt so far away from her; five hours separated us, but it often felt like we were on opposite sides of the earth. I didn't know all of what Aaron's mom and family were telling Eva, but I knew they weren't honest with her.

I remember feeling lonely at my aunt's house. I remember bits and pieces of living there, like scattered puzzle pieces thrown in a pile. Sometimes, I'd try to put them together, never getting much past the edges. I'd find a memory here and there: the fireplace in the living room, the hinged stair in the family room where I hid my toys, the kitchen counter where I ate breakfast with every member of the family.

The memory that stuck with me the most was the smell of Juicy Fruit gum. I was three when I sat on the sunspot in my aunt's hallway by the desk that held the Juicy Fruit gum. I only remember that sunspot because I sat on it every morning, probably for months on end, smelling the gum while my aunt took a shower. I don't think I'd remember anything were it not for the smell. Smells are funny like that. I wonder if Eva remembered her mother's smell. She will be just three when Mommy returns home; will she understand what happened? What will she remember?

My chest is hurting again. I'd better go inside and do something productive. I think I've been sitting too long on this hard branch, and it's affecting my whole body. That's why my chest is hurting. My chest could not be hurting because of my heart—no way. That was fixed!

Chapter 22

UNtimely

My Turn

Memorial Hospital Again!

January 2016

I had my broken heart fixed right before Jessica returned from Holy Cross Hospital. Jack drove the five-hour ride home with me on Sunday. I walked into my cardiologist's office on Monday and announced that I thought there might be something wrong with my heart.

My cardiologist was the kind of guy that would stop everything if he felt you needed him. He was just walking by as I was telling the receptionist that I needed to make an appointment ASAP because I had to go back to Jacksonville.

"Mrs. Thorne!" I heard him before I could see him. "To what do I owe this great honor?" That was Doc, never forgot a face and always made you feel special somehow. "What's wrong?" He asked as he looked me up and down. "You don't look so hot."

"Have her wait a few minutes," he told the receptionist. "I want to see her today."

So, that was it. I sat in his office without an appointment, waiting for Doc to see me for a few minutes. Everyone called him "Doc." One of the most laid-back, unpretentious doctors I ever met, I loved him. I miss him. He passed away just a few months ago. No one will replace him.

Anyway, he saw me that day, and although my EKG was normal, he wanted to do some further testing immediately. He scheduled a stress test for the next day in his office.

I arrived at his office early the next morning and got hooked up to the heart monitor for the test. The first part was the treadmill. I wasn't too worried about the treadmill and assumed I'd pass with flying colors. I still thought all my chest pain was due to the stress of caring for Jessica.

Unfortunately, I didn't last very long on the treadmill, maybe a minute. One minute, my EKG looked good, and I was just walking along without a worry in the world. The next minute, my jaw started hurting. I mentioned it to the technician. She looked at my EKG, which was still normal, but she said we'd better stop since I was having pain.

I had to wait a little while, and then the technician did the nuclear scan of my arteries. I've had lots of medical procedures done over time, and I've become familiar with the way technicians react when everything is fine and when everything is not fine. I could tell that this test fell into the "not fine" category, especially when the technician went running out of the room to find the doctor.

It wasn't long after the technician sprinted out of the room that Doc was on the phone with Jack. I didn't know it was Jack he was talking to, but I overheard him saying, "...either you come right away and take her to the emergency room, or we'll call an ambulance!"

At this point, I was calmly sitting in the nuclear stress test waiting room watching everyone in Doc's office run around like chickens with their heads cut off.

Wow, someone must be really sick. I thought to myself. I still didn't think it concerned me since I was told to sit in the waiting room.

"Where's the CD?" Doc was barking at the technician that performed my test. "I can't hold," he screamed into the phone. "I need to talk to him now. I'm sending a patient to the hospital, and he needs to see her immediately!"

"Doc." The technician was waving the CD in his face.

I finally realized that all the commotion was about me when Jack was ushered into the waiting room, and Doc told him to take me to the hospital immediately.

A half-hour later, I arrived at the same hospital where Jessica spent almost a month in the ICU. Jack dropped me off at the front of the ER and went to park the car. I don't think either one of us realized the seriousness of the situation.

I walked into the emergency room, gave the lady my name, information, and handed her the CD. The staff immediately rushed me to triage, ahead of the 50 or so people sitting in the waiting room. A nurse bearing a striking resemblance to Nurse Ratched from "One Flew over the Cuckoo's Nest" ordered me onto a gurney and informed me that I'd be getting undressed for surgery.

"Surgery," I cried. "Why do I need surgery?" I started taking off my clothes.

"No," Ratched's lipstick-stained teeth yelled at me. "I'll be taking off your clothes in a moment after the doctor comes in and explains the surgery."

At that moment, a man wearing breathtaking leather cowboy boots appeared behind Nurse Ratched. She left; he stepped forward. I envied his boots.

"Nice boots," I commented.

"Thanks," he said. "I'm Dr. Aaberg, and I'll be doing your catheterization and stents."

I guess my blank stare gave him a hint that I had no clue what he was talking about.

"You shouldn't be alive right now." He patted my arm. "You have five blockages in your heart. One of the blockages you have is called the 'widowmaker' because it usually happens to men, and it kills them very suddenly. Your main artery into your heart is 95% blocked. I've never had a patient 'walk' into the emergency room with the kinds of blockages you have. I'm going to get ready now. You'll be sedated, but not asleep. I'll see you in a few minutes." He left.

I listened to his cowboy boots click down the hall for a very long time. They say that the sense of hearing is the last thing to go. I hoped everything else was working as well as my ears when I saw Ratched out of the corner of my eye.

Ratched didn't say a word to me as she started pulling off my clothing with surprising finesse. I was naked and shivering in less than three seconds. The delightful hospital gown and slippers followed, and I was given a threadbare cover, which did little to ease the shivering.

Ratched wasn't big on pleasantries. "Anyone with you?" she asked.

"Yes," I replied. "My husband is in the waiting room."

"I'll get him," she said as she left.

Jack met me in the hall as I was being wheeled into surgery. My brain was swimming in a deep fog from the anesthesia coursing through my veins. I managed a thin smile in his direction. "Guess you're not going to be a widower today," I said.

"I love you," he replied as he kissed me goodbye.

What kind of bye are we talking about here? I was considering all the goodbyes I didn't say to my kids etc. when the bright light of the operating room came into focus, and my brain went out of focus.

I don't know how long "Dr. Cowboy Boots" spent with me in the operating room because I drifted in and out of consciousness. All I know is that he looked exhausted when he came to see me shortly after the procedure.

"Well, that was fun," he said. "You're lucky to be alive!"

"You already told me that," I managed a weak reply. "I still like your boots."

"Thank you." He continued, "I was only able to fix three out of five blockages today. You still have two blockages that we'll have to fix later. It took a lot longer than expected."

"Did I have a heart attack?" I still didn't know what had happened to me.

"Surprisingly, no." He pulled out a picture of my arteries taken during the procedure. "This is your heart." I remember thinking about the stupid commercial that says, "This is your brain. This is your brain on drugs," and a frying egg appears. My brain was on a lot of drugs, so it didn't stick around for long. I don't remember what else Dr. Cowboy Boots said or when he left.

So, I guess I didn't have a heart attack after all. It seems I was a walking miracle. I didn't have a heart attack, but I did end up having something else happen to me while I was still in the hospital—a brain aneurysm!

Chapter 23

UNexpected

Home at Last

Day 80
By Jack

Originally Gwen was going to do this next update. She has a passion and skill for writing that I will never come close to. Unfortunately, Gwen is still in the hospital recovering from heart and brain issues. She is getting better, but the bleed to her brain affected her cerebellum, which controls her balance and coordination. This has caused her to feel that the room is spinning every time she attempts to stand or sit-up. We're not out of the woods yet, but I think she'll be home soon and be able to continue to play a big part in Jessica's recovery.

The big news is that Jess came home today! She was finally united with her baby after two and a half long months. This reunion has continuously been on her mind, and now that she has finally been reunited with Eva, I think her recovery will shift into a whole other gear. Jess has come a long way but still has a long road ahead of her. The left side of her body is still struggling from the stroke, but she is a true warrior and will continue to fight back.

Last Monday, Emily and I went to Jacksonville and watched as they put Jessica's left arm through a series of range of motion movements. It was so painful that she was in tears, but never was there a thought of quitting or stopping. I think back to where Jess was at the beginning of this journey and truly am amazed at her achievement. A large part of her progress is due to the tremendous support she has received from a wide variety of people. As I mentioned earlier, we still have a long road ahead of us, and your support and prayers will still be needed.

Memorial Hospital Again

The heart catheterization with stents was supposed to be a fairly routine surgery. However, I never do anything routine. My motto is: "Always keep them guessing," or maybe it's: "Never a dull moment."

In any case, I ended up with the same doctor Jessica had because my body decided a brain bleed was just the thing I needed to muddy the waters. One minute I was sitting in bed playing cards with Emily, and the next moment I was puking my brains out and hoping to die.

The headache was unbearable. It came on so suddenly that I had no time to react. All I remember is uncontrollable puking. The projectile vomit hurled across the room, missing Emily by a few inches. It just kept on coming as I held my head and moaned in agony. Emily ran out and got the nurse who called some kind of code, and my room quickly filled with doctors and nurses hustling and bustling all around. Emily was ushered out of the room, and I was rushed to ICU.

I imagine my headache was very much the same as Jessica's headache when she had the brain bleed. Maybe this was God's way of telling me what my daughter must have experienced. I don't remember much of what happened next. I heard bits and pieces of conversations between Dr. Cowboy Boots and Jessica's doctor...ventilator, surgery, stop the bleeding, medicine for vomiting—I remember saying, "No ventilator."

Then, the nurse gave me something in my IV, and I quickly stopped puking and fell asleep.

When I awoke, I felt much better. Emily, Jack, Lucy, and a few of my friends were keeping vigil in my room. I tried to sit up, but the room started spinning, and I closed my eyes again. No one knew I was awake. I heard them talking. (They say hearing is the last sense to go). Jack was saying something about staying in the hospital for two more weeks, and Emily was saying that probably wasn't going to be enough time.

Enough time for what? I thought as I drifted away.

I fell back asleep. I dreamt about an angel in my room, standing on top of my IV pole. The angel was spinning around like a ballerina, and her sparkling wings were making little lights shine all over the room like tiny fireflies. It was beautiful and so peaceful.

I wanted to stay in the dream. I wanted to join the angel in her dance. I wanted to fly away with her. I didn't fly away, though.

I woke up to a tolerable headache, and instead of a spinning angel, a spinning husband.

"Why are you spinning?" I asked.

"I'm not," he replied.

"Yes, you are. You're spinning, and so is everything in the room," I snapped.

"You had a brain bleed in your balance center, and that's why everything seems like it's spinning," he said in his matter-of-fact style.

"Oh, that explains it," I growled. "Thanks for being so understanding!"

I don't know what I expected from Jack at that moment. Did I expect him to pour out his feelings and tell me he was so glad I didn't make him a widower? That wasn't Jack. Jack wasn't a hopeless romantic. Jack wasn't the kind of guy that would set out a rose petal trail to the bedroom. Jack was more likely to blaze a path through the flea market and tell me to keep up with him. I even wrote a story or two about his love of flea markets: Flea Guy paints a great picture of Jack.

Reflection

It's important to note that the sudden onset of a severe headache or WHOL (worst headache of life) is a common symptom of a brain aneurysm.

Chapter 24

UNconventional

Flea Guy

If my husband Jack had his own TV show, it would be called Flea Guy because he is a flea market junkie. Or maybe, more accurately, a garage sale fanatic. I swear, he can smell a garage sale from five miles away, and the car must have some secret built-in radar system. Call me a conspiracy theorist, but I believe that there is a group of them out there with their radios tuned to a special station that picks up the radar. You can spot them in their cars, scanning the medians for the bleeding garage sale signs with the obscured arrows.

They're the ones that'll do donuts on a dime in the middle of a congested highway, pull up to the curbside, leave their cars running and block five lanes of traffic. They race out of their vehicles, skim the contents of a driveway in the blink of an eye, purchase a gold necklace buried in the bottom of a pile of shells, and sprint back to the car in ten seconds flat. Jack has been known to dash to the next thrift store or garage sale before he realizes that he left me two garage sales back.

When we go together to flea markets, it's much worse. I've decided that I need my own Segway to keep up with Jack. At the flea market, he's the ten-speed bike, and I'm the three-wheel trike. He's always leaving me in his dust, which is why I don't feel a bit guilty about the pair of shrunken heads I purchased in his absence. Anyway, he is the master of the bargain. While my fifty dollar shrunken heads sit in the garage freaking out all the neighborhood kids and giving them nightmares, his ten-cent book sells on the internet for four hundred dollars. He is amazing.

Not only does my husband haunt garage sales, flea markets, and auctions, but he also frequents thrift stores. Once, for his birthday, I made up personal gift certificates for him and delivered them to the local thrift stores. Then I gave him a map with clues and sent him on his *own* scavenger hunt from one thrift store to another. It was pure genius (if I do say so myself).

Jack and I have been married for twenty-five years, and I don't believe he's ever missed a Saturday morning garage sale or flea market. On one road trip from Florida to New Jersey with the kids (in the truck with the missing back window), he took a small detour and arrived at his favorite flea market a tad early, 3 a.m. It was frigid cold, so he bundled the kids in blankets and told them to get some shut-eye before the flea market opened at five. Needless to say, that is one memory etched into the fabric of our family forever. There's another memory that I'm reminded of every time I walk into my closet.

I admit that I am not a "cleaner outer." When I hang something in the back of my closet, it is because I don't plan on wearing it for at least the next ten years, but I keep it just in case I lose that extra twenty pounds. Anyway, something must have come over me about five years ago when I made a valiant attempt to declutter my side of the bulging mess that we call a walk-in closet. It is more like a "trip-in" closet due to the vast array of mismatched shoes and other sundries littering the closet floor.

Anyway, as I was saying, I was a decluttering queen. I showed no mercy to the blouses screaming that I only had fifteen pounds to go, the tie-dyed jeans that reminded me they were coming back in fashion, or the argyle sweaters growing dust bunnies. They all got squished into the dreaded thrift store garbage bag where old clothes gasp their last breath.

So, as I said, my husband has been known to haunt a few thrift stores from time to time. Usually, when he returns home, he brings me out to the car to dazzle me with his finds. He is always very considerate of my latest undertaking and frequently brings back some fantastic one-of-a-kind treasure to enhance my project. Once, he brought me an entire frog band made from recycled metal for my garden.

A few months after I cleaned out my closet, he was off on one of his shopping sprees. This time, when he returned home, he was especially proud of his find.

"Honey, you're not going to believe what I found!" he said breathlessly as he grabbed my hand and pulled me to the car. He was so excited, like a kid in a candy shop. I couldn't imagine what he found that excited him so. He even made me close my eyes.

You can imagine my surprise when I was finally allowed to open my eyes and behold the treasure. There, right in front of me, stood my husband grinning from ear to ear, holding a familiar item.

"Can you believe it?" he laughed. "I found a blouse just like the one you used to wear when we were first married."

I was speechless! There it was in all its 1980s glory, my old blouse that might cover one boob now if I positioned it just so.

"Oh, honey," I crooned, "How did you ever find the exact same blouse?"

"I know, right?" he grinned. "Amazing, huh?"

I just couldn't bear to tell him the truth. I couldn't admit to him that I had just sent that blouse to the thrift store during my cleaning frenzy. So, I lovingly took the blouse, kissed my husband, and thanked him for his incredible find.

Some women have husbands that bring them diamond rings. Some women have husbands that wine and dine them and cover their pillows in rose petals, but I bet that I am the only woman who has a husband who not only remembers what I wore twenty years ago but believes that I can still fit in it!

I made my way to the closet and hung the blouse on the very same hanger it vacated just about a month earlier. I don't know, but I think I might have heard it chuckle (kind of like the last laugh) as I placed it back in its empty spot in the closet.

Jack

When Jack wasn't showering me with flea market/thrift store gifts, he was throwing a mattress in the back of his pickup truck and parking in a swanky hotel parking lot so he could tell everyone we spent the night in the Marriott by the Sea. True, we spent the night, but it was far from the luxury suite. I miss those nights of lying in the back of the pickup truck looking up at the stars, playing scrabble, drinking beer and laughing at our little secret parking lot spot.

Perhaps we're not staying at the Marriott these days, but now that we are older and less comfortable in the back of a pickup truck, Jack has upgraded our hotel experience. I wrote a story about a recent stay at the Cadillac Hotel.

My husband likes to stretch a dollar. Some might even call him cheap or a tightwad. When we travel, he loves to shop around for budget hotels. Before a trip, he'll get those hotel coupon magazines that you see in all the truck stops and scour them for amazing deals.

He's managed to traumatize all of our children with creepy hotels. For instance, there was the time when we were walking into a hotel, and Lucy innocently asked her father why the two men were sitting on the curb drinking out of brown paper bags, and he replied, "I'm sure they are very nice men."

Then there was the time when I was fast asleep but had this strange sensation that someone was staring at me. I opened one eye to see Jessica, Emily, and Lucy standing over me, all staring at my forehead. Jessica yelled, "Don't move, Mom!"

I ask you, what does one do when three children are standing over you while you're sleeping and then one of them shouts?

"Don't move, Mom!"

I didn't just move, I screamed, bolted out of bed and ran out of the room butt naked. Apparently, there was a cockroach the size of Godzilla crawling over my face, and the girls were trying to figure out how to kill it without waking me.

That wasn't our only "critter" experience. There was the close encounter with the rat running across the bed and some other incidents that were so traumatizing, I think I've blocked them from memory. But there is one hotel hellhole that trumps all the others by far. Let me say that I have not embellished this story one iota. It is told exactly as it happened.

O.K. Corral

About five years ago, Jack was playing on a men's tennis team, and they made it to the finals, which were being played on Longboat Key Island about three hours from our house. Jack told me not to worry about a thing because he booked us a room at the Cadillac Hotel. The Cadillac hotel sounded like a nice place to me. Besides, it was on a resort island, so I figured it had to be okay.

What Jack failed to tell me was that the hotel wasn't actually "on" the island. It was "close" to the island. The rest of the team and their wives (except one single guy) were staying "on" the island close to the tournament location.

As we were getting close to the resort island, Jack handed me the page he tore from one of his coupon books.

"You didn't tell me the Cadillac Hotel was in the coupon book," I said as my red alert radar began to kick in.

"Oh, didn't I?" he replied innocently. "Just tell me the address."

I looked at the torn page and found the postage stamp ad for the Cadillac hotel in the bottom left corner.

"I need a magnifying glass to read this," I complained. I got out my high-powered reading glasses.

"Oh, here's the address under the beautiful picture of the concrete pool," I said as the sarcasm oozed from my voice, "1117 MLK Boulevard."

"Look, we're only staying one night, and Joe's staying there too," Jack said as he turned off the road leading to the island and headed for downtown.

"That's supposed to make me feel better!" I retorted. "Joe is so cheap he usually sleeps in the back of his truck in the hotel parking lots."

"Well," Jack said, "Aren't we getting hoity-toity. Have you forgotten that we used to do the same thing when we were first married?"

Okay, maybe we did throw the mattress in the back of the pickup and stay in the Marriott By the Sea parking lot a few times, but that's when we were broke, and it was sort of romantic back then. Now, we could afford to stay in a halfway decent place, but I was tired, and there were no other hotels in the area since this was the tourist season.

So, I gave in, and we found the Cadillac Hotel in a rundown section of town just across the street from the Salvation Army thrift store (I don't believe that was just a coincidence). I'd be willing to bet that Jack did a Google search for hotels within five miles of thrift stores. We'd hardly checked in, and he was out the door and on his way across the street.

While he was gone, I decided to check out the concrete pool. It was concrete alright—and empty. I returned to the room and turned on the air conditioner, which was loud enough to wake the dead. Things started looking up when I discovered that the TV worked and even got four channels. The highlight of the Cadillac Hotel was the refrigerator in each room. Our fridge also came stocked—leftover Chinese food and half a beer.

"It doesn't get any better than this," I said, pointing to the leftovers as Jack returned from his Salvation Army jaunt.

"Look, let's just sleep here tonight, and we'll find a different place in the morning," he said as he covered the bed with a blanket from our car.

Luckily, Jack and I had brought our pillows, so we slept fully clothed on top of the blanket from our car. Surprisingly, we both slept soundly through the night. I don't know if it was the loud drone of the air conditioner or the mental exhaustion, but not even the sounds of the gunfight woke us up!

So, the next morning I woke up early and decided to take a stroll down MLK Blvd., but my walk was cut short when I opened my door to the crime scene tape stretched around the corner room of the Cadillac hotel.

"What in God's name..." I started to say as my eyes took in the scene.

I kid you not, sticking out of the corner room of the Cadillac hotel beyond the crime scene tape was a mangled Cadillac.

"Jack!" I yelled as I ran over to the bed and shook my husband, "wake up. There's a Cadillac stuck in a hotel room."

"What?" He said drowsily, "it is the Cadillac hotel."

"No," I shouted, "it wasn't there yesterday, and there's crime scene tape!"

"Okay, okay." He stood. "Let's go see what happened."

The hotel clerk seemed unfazed by the crime scene tape. He calmly explained that, sometime during the night, the person who was involved in the high-speed police chase down MLK Blvd. decided to check his Caddy into the Cadillac hotel and proceed on foot behind the hotel (right behind our room).

A gunfight ensued, and the wounded perp tried to run back to his Caddy (which would explain the bloodstains all over the parking lot). He tried to make his getaway, but the car wasn't budging from its room, and the guy was subsequently arrested.

The bored clerk then asked, "So, will you be staying with us another night?"

"No," I replied as I handed him my keys. "My husband booked us a room at the O.K. Corral for tonight."

Reflection

This is what I know to be true about Jack: The one who loves you will never leave you because, even if there are 100 reasons to give up, he will find one reason to hold on.

Over this past year, I knew he was holding on, maybe by his fingernails, but he was still holding on. I was grateful for that. I was also thankful for his steady presence. I don't think I told him that enough. I mostly just got frustrated with him because I wanted him to fix everything. I wanted him to ride in on his fancy steed (from our farm), guns blazing to rescue me. Never mind that Jack never rode a horse or shot a firearm or even wore cowboy boots in his entire life. In fact, Jack never wanted to live on a farm.

Chapter 25

UNwinding

Day 97

God's Got This

February 6, 2016

Jessica had an angiogram of the brain done on Thursday, and it went well. Here is what Aaron posted on Facebook about the procedure:

"God is great! Jess's procedure went well, and the aneurysm that was coiled in October is not filling with blood at all. The next step is to clip the other aneurysm, which hasn't changed or gotten worse and replace the skull flap. At this point, we don't know when that will happen, but her doctor said within the month. Thank you again for all the prayers."

I spoke with Jess on the phone, and she sounded well. My own health story continued. I saw the neurosurgeon for an update, (the same one Jess sees), and he had some good news.

"You don't have to worry about the brain bleed, and you should be less dizzy and have fewer headaches within the next two months."

As for my heart, it was very broken in so many ways. I would get rather tired just from walking and doing regular things around the house. Well, I had to use a walker to get around the house, and I had to concentrate fully on not falling over when I walked, so I hadn't been doing regular things around the house. Regular things would be folding laundry, dishes, vacuuming, etc. Those regular things I left for Jack and Lucy. I was lucky if I could walk from my couch to my office without having exhaustion overwhelm me.

This tiredness could have been from the brain bleed or from the 80% blockage I still had in my heart. I simply didn't know at that point. I looked forward to seeing Doc the following Monday and Dr. Cowboy Boots, the heart surgeon, at the end of the month. I knew they wanted to correct the blockage at some point, but it was a high-risk procedure because of the blood thinners I had to be on due to the stents that they already put in. So, my heart remained broken.

Nowadays, a broken heart should be fixed easily. I hoped that was the case with my mechanical heart that beat in my chest. As far as my emotional heart goes, it was not such an easy fix. I realized that I had to put many of my dreams on the back burner, or maybe give up on them. I realized that my life had been forever altered in so many ways—altered or shattered. I'm not sure which word fits best.

On a positive note, I was listening to Joel Osteen, and he was speaking about what it means to be rich. I listened to him describing a "rich" man who had a beautiful house, lots of money and many cars. Then, of course, he went on to talk about the real meaning of rich. Riches come in all shapes and sizes.

I was rich with my family and friends. I had riches in my five-acre farm and home: horses to watch, chickens that gave us eggs, roosters that woke me in the morning, and beautiful oaks to sit under. I hoped that I was rich in faith. I hoped that my faith would give me the strength to believe that God had a brilliant and mighty plan for all of these current trials. I prayed that my faith would see me through and that Jess would once again be an integral part of our family's lives. This is what I had to believe: God's got this, doesn't he?

Chapter 26

UNfed

The Farm

December 2016

So now, as I sit under the oaks, my heart is hurting again, or I think it might be my heart. I'll go back to the cardiologist—just to get it checked. Unfortunately, the new doctor is nothing like Doc. The guy who took Doc's place is stern, stoic, and detached, but Doc hired him before he died from cancer, and I trust Doc's judgment. I also trust Doc's staff. They're all still there, and they've known me for over ten years. They take care of me there, and I find comfort in that fact. I'll make the appointment tomorrow.

I've been on this branch for a long time. I'm going to change my perch to my computer inside. It's by the window where I can look out at the miniature donkeys and sit in the A/C. I might even put the lobster in boiling water for Lucy when I go in. I'm sure she hasn't done it yet.

The donkeys spot me on my way back to the house. They announce that I still haven't fed them, so I detour to the barn. The smell of hay hits me first, followed by the smell of horse manure and donkey. I'll try to describe donkey smell, musty maybe mixed with dank. I love these smells, don't know why. Still, they bring me peace.

I feed all of the animals: hay to Wilma and Pebbles, the donkeys, and Felix, the horse. I feed Roo Roo, the rooster, and all the chickens (too many to name), and I give a bone to our barn dog, Fred. My work here is done—time to kill a lobster.

"Mom," Lucy heard the front door open. "Please!" She was holding the lobster and trying to cut off the rubber bands that were keeping its claws from opening.

The lobster looked like it was winning this battle and was about to escape Lucy's grasp. I laughed. She didn't. I got the teenage stink eye and knew that Lucy was at wit's end with the lobster.

"Is the water boiling?" I calmly asked.

"Yes," came her exasperated reply. "It's been boiling." Eye roll.

"Okay," I said. "Do you have scissors?"

"Yes." Another eye roll followed by tears. "I wanted to do this by myself."

"It's okay, Lucy. Why don't I hold the lobster, and you cut off the rubber bands?" I said in my "mother knows best" voice.

I gingerly took the lobster from her grasp and told her to pick up the scissors. She cut off the rubber bands, and I plunged the writhing lobster headfirst into the large pot of boiling water. Lucy's screams mixed with the lobster's as she ran out of the kitchen.

"Set the timer," I yelled at her as I made my way to the computer room.

This is my birthday dinner, after all. Do I have to do all the cooking?

By now, I've spun my yarn until it is almost as big as the world's largest ball of twine, which weighs 19,873 pounds. (This is not a factoid that I know off the top of my head. I looked it up.)

As I unravel my tale, it occurs to me that it has taken 58 years to spin this yarn. The world's biggest ball of twine has five more years on me since it was started in 1953. It weighs more than my ball of twine, but I think my yarn is more interesting.

Spinning my yarn isn't always easy. It's not easy to explain why I have a black daughter and a Muslim daughter. It's not easy to tell the story of my oldest daughter, Jessica, or the story of my son, Kevin. So, I will do my best to relate how it all happened.

I started this story with Jessica's brain aneurysm and stroke, but there was an entire life leading up to that day. Like I said earlier, this story is a 1000-piece puzzle with only the edges of the puzzle pieces completed thus far. I feel like I have to add the rest of the puzzle pieces now.

I'm not sure how to add the rest of the pieces, so I'll just stick to the facts like Dragnet. "The facts, ma'am, just the facts."

Chapter 27

Unspoken

Early '60s Late '70s

In the Beginning

I already explained that my mom died. She died at home on the couch. I guess she may have had a brain bleed (since they tend to run in families), and no one knew back then what had happened. I've heard from my aunt and grandmother that she had a headache, and I'm assuming her chest was hurting, so she lay down on the couch. If it was a heart attack and myocarditis (an infection in her heart) as the autopsy stated with some uncertainty, it killed her instantly.

My mom died, and my dad moved the family to my aunt's house. I suppose a lot more pieces of the puzzle were added at that time, but I was too young to remember, and no one ever felt the necessity to tell the kids what really happened. We didn't even go to the funeral, or so I heard over the years from various people. I went through a stage of asking questions, but I quickly learned that children were to be seen and not heard.

Children with dead mothers should never be heard! Children with dead mothers needed to be protected from the truth at all costs. Dead mothers never existed in the first place. She didn't die after all; she just disappeared. She went to the store and never came back.

All of her pictures, all of her treasured belongings, all of her clothes—everything that defined her, or her existence, went to the store with her. She took it all. Nothing was left except for a few vague memories in the far recesses of people's minds, I guess. I couldn't access the recesses of those minds, though—God knows I tried.

Once, I made the mistake of asking my dad about her. His answer: "She was just like you."

What the heck did that mean? Just like me. Stubborn? Was she stubborn? I'm stubborn. Strong-willed? I'm strong-willed. Athletic? I'm athletic. Did she love animals? I love animals, except when they're begging to be fed, and I have to clean up their messes. Did we look alike? I didn't know. There were no pictures. So many questions spun in my head. They were never answered.

I couldn't get the follow-up question out of my mouth fast enough. I wasn't a lawyer, after all. I was an eight-year-old girl asking about a mother that had been Mr. Cleaned, Cloroxed, and Windexed out of my life. If I had a follow-up question, it fell on deaf ears as my dad made his hasty retreat. "What kind of 'just like you' are we talking about here?"

I never knew. I never knew what "just like you" meant, and I never asked my dad again.

I asked my grandmother and my aunt about my mother. They filled in the blanks a little bit, but not much. I heard a story about how my mom once wore my aunt's shoes to march in a parade, and the shoes disintegrated. I learned that my mom did, in fact, love animals and tried to bring a cat home once that she had found in a phone booth. I learned that my mom used to work for the telephone company, but I don't know what she did. She also was an outstanding bowler. Where I heard that is still a mystery to me.

Once, when I was a teenager (I'm not sure how old I was), my sister snuck my brother and me into a room on Christmas Day. Under a shroud of darkness (or so it seemed), she handed each of us our Christmas present. It was a picture of my mom! It was the only picture I ever saw of my mom, a portrait. My mom was beautiful. I don't even know where my sister found the picture, and I didn't ask.

Years later, I displayed the picture in my home. I felt like I was breaking some unspoken, but terribly important, family rule. I was sure that I would suffer a horrible familial consequence for such a blatant display of my mother. No one ever said anything about the picture. It still has a prominent spot in my home, and I'm forever grateful that my sister thought enough to give me such a precious gift.

Perhaps it's the profound loss I suffered at such a young age that prompted me to place motherhood at the top of my "most honorable professions" list. Whatever the reason, I vowed early on in my life that I would strive to be the best mom I could.

I wanted to elevate motherhood to superhero status singlehandedly. Never mind that I needed the assistance of a father figure to fulfill this dream. I knew in my heart that I would be a great mom, and I planned on having at least ten kids.

What's that old Yiddish proverb? "Man plans, and God laughs?" I'm sure God was laughing as I made my plans for so many kids.

Reflection

Speaking of Yiddish proverbs, I came up with a few Yiddish curses for Aaron. I'm not really going to curse him, but I was tempted.

"May you grow like an onion with your head in the ground."

"May your bones be broken as often as the Ten Commandments."

"May you eat chopped liver with onions, *shmaltz* herring, chicken soup with dumplings, baked carp with horseradish, braised meat with vegetable stew, latkes, tea with lemon, every day—and may you choke on every bite!" (I think I'll add, "and may you gain 600 lbs." to that one.)

"May God help you like cupping helps a corpse."

"May he become swollen and veined like a mountain."

"Salt in his eyes and pepper in his nose! A boil in his throat!"

"May all your teeth fall out, except one to give you a toothache."

"May you have thunder in your belly and lightning in your pants."

"God should visit upon him the best of the ten plagues."

But I digress.

Chapter 28

Unpacking

1980s

Florida

Our move to Florida was a bit of a surprise. In May, Jack got a phone call from a school in Dade County, offering him a teaching/coaching position starting in late August. He took the job without seeing the school. We were young and foolish enough to think that we could simply move to Dade County without a clue as to where it was or where we would live. We sold our house, rented a U-Haul, packed up the truck and car (one-year-old Jess in her car seat), and off we went.

The 20-hour drive was grueling, mainly because I was driving the car with Jess in the backseat, and Jack was ahead of me in the truck pulling the U-Haul. We didn't have cell phones back then, and he was too far ahead of me to beep my horn, so I couldn't get his attention when we needed to stop.

Jack has tunnel vision when he gets behind the wheel for a long trip and the bladder of the world's largest camel. I don't know if he had a secret supply of no-doze in his glove compartment, but he started driving and never looked back. The only thing that kept me awake during this godawful drive were thoughts of strangling Jack the next time we stopped for gas.

Stopping for gas should have been an easy endeavor.

It wasn't.

Did I mention that neither Jack nor I can back up a truck with a trailer attached?

The "backing up" episode occurred around 10 p.m. when we were both exhausted, and Jess was wet and miserable. Jack had finally pulled off the highway for gas, and I ran to the restroom while he was fueling up.

When I came out of the bathroom, I noticed Jack was surveying the parking lot, looking for the exit. Unfortunately, this exit required one of us to back up the truck with the trailer.

"We have to back the truck up," Jack informed me as I was changing Jess in the back seat.

"Okay," I said, "what's the problem?"

"I keep backing it up wrong," Jack admitted. "I almost hit the pump twice."

"Do you want me to try?" I asked

"Yes," he said. "I'll direct you."

I got behind the wheel and proceeded to back up.

"Turn the tires!" He began yelling at me. "You're going to run into the pump."

"Don't yell at me!" I shouted. "Which way should I turn the damn tires?"

"Left!" he screamed. "Turn them left."

I did. The trailer went closer to the pump.

We must have looked like a Laurel and Hardy comedy routine trying to move our U-Haul. Finally, a trucker, who took pity on us, came over and got the truck/trailer to the exit. We thanked him profusely. I begged Jack to find a hotel so we could all get some rest.

An hour later, I pulled the car into a hotel parking lot to survey the layout so Jack would not have to back up anymore. It looked okay to me, so I told him to pull in.

Oops....

We went to check in and were told that there were no more rooms. I wanted to slap the clerk, but we left before I made a fool of myself.

I got in the car. Jack got in the truck. I started toward the exit and realized that the parking lot did not have a way through. Jack was behind me, honking at me to get moving.

I got out of the car and walked back to the truck.

"There's no exit at this end," I said wearily. "You'll have to back out."

"What?" Jack looked like he was going to explode. "I can't back this thing out."

We went back into the office. Surprisingly, the clerk said there was one room that was handicapped accessible, which she was supposed to keep open for anyone who is handicapped.

"We're handicapped," I said. "We cannot back up a truck with a trailer, and we are currently in the middle of your parking lot, blocking about half your customers."

She gave us the room.

In the morning, Jack had to wait in the parking lot for the people to move their cars. It was awful. There were so many cars and so many people who wanted to get on the road. Jack had to move the truck up and back (just enough to let people out) until he could finally pull it up into a parking space. It was noon before there was enough room in the parking lot to get the truck out.

I think we were in Georgia at that time. I don't remember. All I know is we had at least ten more hours of driving. I tried to make Jack understand that he needed to pay closer attention to my car behind him.

"If I'm blinking my lights at you, please find a place to stop," I begged.

Later, I was madly blinking my lights as I was slapping myself in the face trying to stay awake. Jess was sound asleep in the backseat as my car swerved on and off the road. Jack was oblivious to my plight. He just kept right on going. Needless to say, when we stopped for gas, I was no longer talking to him. Later, when the truck got stuck in the marsh with the alligators converging, I didn't even open my mouth. I just got in the car and drove Jess and me out of danger.

I don't know how we made it to our destination without killing each other or killing ourselves by running off the road or being eaten by hungry alligators. When we finally arrived in Dade County, we had to find a place to stay.

I had a friend who lived nearby and offered her home for a short time. We stayed with her for two weeks until we found a long-term hotel. The hotel was home for the next two weeks until we moved into an apartment, but it all worked out in the end. We've been in Florida for 29 years now.

Over those 29 years, we've experienced a lot of joy and heartache. Perhaps the most devastating disappointment of all is the fact that I had six miscarriages. It's one of the reasons why Jack and I decided that we should become foster parents. I wrote a story about the miscarriages after I heard a very poignant song, "Carry You" by Selah.

Carry You

It was April 20, 1989, when my heart ached with emptiness. I felt so hollow inside on that day, just like all the other days. Now, so many years later, something comes along to trigger the memory, and the pain wells up like a newly formed wound that feels like it will take forever to heal all over again. The wound from 1989 has left a huge scar for sure. Scarred, that is how I felt back then—scarred for life. Scarred about life and scarred from life.

That day, it was a song: "I Will Carry You." I started the day, asking God to answer my whispered prayer. I didn't expect him to rip open an old wound.

"Is that really how you answer prayer, God? Thanks a lot!"

Why? Why that day of all days, did God allow me to read that story and listen to that song that brought years of mourning into this morning: This regular everyday morning when I was just going about my everyday business praying my everyday prayers?

Six. That is the magic number. Six babies. Six little souls. Six massive gaping wounds. The one wound from April 20, 1989, is the "gapiest" I guess. It's that way because the others were so young. They barely made it to three months old. Hardly a baby, after all. I did feel them, though. I felt them stir. Maybe I just imagined it, but I know in my heart and soul they were a part of me.

God blessed me with them. He asked me to carry them. I told Him I would. Then, like some mean, hateful revengeful...I don't know; he took them away.

All of them.

Does God empty you completely so that He can fill you up again? Is that what He was doing? God sure did a thorough job of emptying me. He emptied me of my joy when He emptied my soul. He emptied my uterus. I didn't love Him then. I didn't trust Him then. I didn't turn to Him then. I didn't want any part of Him then. I wanted my babies. They were mine!

The first five were barely a flicker in my eye. The doctors were so cavalier about the whole thing. "Oh," they'd say, "there had to be something terribly wrong with the baby. It's nature's way of taking care of things." Nature's way. Really? Every time I'd leave each doctor's office feeling entirely empty, I couldn't explain the void to anyone. Not to my husband. Not to my family or friends. Not to God.

I'm not going to lie. I'm not going to sugar coat this. I'm not going to say that I didn't scream and cry and shout and raise my fist to the heavens and curse the God that asked me to be the mother to these precious souls and then cruelly snatched them out of my life. I had no one. No one understood my pain. No one understood my loss. No one understood the depths of my emptiness. Not them and not God.

The one I remember most was the one that made it past three months. That one was going to make it all the way. I just knew it. And then...again, I experienced the sinkhole, the bottomless pit of sorrow and longing for something lost, but not forgotten. I never had closure—no funeral to mourn the loss, no friends and family surrounding me in my time of sorrow. "It" was not a "real baby" after all. It wasn't born; it was just lost.

I hated it when people referred to my child as "it." My baby was not an "it." My baby was a child in my womb, growing and waiting to enter the world. My baby had a heartbeat and a soul and a future. He or she was a unique human being; a one of a kind person that God created. I couldn't wait to bring this glorious child into the world. Then, inexplicably, the baby was "lost."

"I didn't 'lose the baby," I wanted to scream. "The baby is still with me," I wanted to shout to the unheeding world.

Yet, I didn't shout, didn't scream; I quietly mourned alone.

Later, I finally allowed my fingers to play the rhythm of the story, the baby's story—our family's story. The story that yearned to be born; the story that poured from my salty ocean of tears; the story of the tidal wave:

Life is like the ocean's waves. Most times, the waves are predictable like clockwork, ebbing and flowing in a steady rhythm. Then, there are the times of restless choppiness when the rhythm is interrupted, and the waves crash to shore in angry bursts.

Finally, there is the tidal wave, which sweeps in and changes the entire landscape in one fell swoop.

The longer we live, the more we come to realize that the steady rhythm of our lives can become choppy in an instant. Often, tidal waves come out of nowhere and change the entire way you look at the terrain of your life.

As the waves etch their presence into the sandy shore, so do the waves of our lives carve our faces.

Our wrinkles are life's roadmap. Each one has a story and a memory attached to it. Wouldn't it be wonderful if we could just touch a "smile" wrinkle and relive the moment that etched it into our face? Sometimes, we do feel a wrinkle in a roundabout way. That is what happened to me when I heard that song, "Carry You."

Unfortunately, it wasn't a smile wrinkle; it was a tidal wave wrinkle.

It was a real baby, I heard my mind screaming as the tears streamed down my face and flowed over the crevices formed in April of 1989.

April ushered in a beautiful, sunny weekend. Jack and I planned to have a picnic with Jess. We had some projects planned as well, so I decided to get a head start on one of them, refinishing a coffee table. I began sanding the table when, without warning, I felt a sharp pain in my abdomen.

I was five months pregnant, so the pain concerned me more than usual. Shortly after feeling the pain, I started spotting. I called the doctor, who did not seem to be too alarmed. He tried to reassure me as he told me to rest over the weekend. He said I could wait until Monday to make an appointment. I wasn't reassured. I was terrified.

It was the longest weekend of my life! We did not go on our picnic. I stayed off my feet, trying to read or watch TV, but nothing was penetrating my paralyzed brain. Jack, Jess, and I spent many hours praying that our baby was going to be okay. As the weekend dragged on, I kept second-guessing my decision to start refinishing the coffee table. Did I do something wrong that hurt the baby? Did I move the wrong way? Did I breathe some toxic dust?

By the time Monday rolled around, I was a basket case. Jack asked if I wanted him to go to the appointment with me. I told him to go to work even though my heart was screaming, "I need you to go with me!" On some level, I resented the fact that he even had to ask, so I dug in my stubborn heels and pretended that I could handle this alone.

I drove to the doctor's office in a fog. I kept telling myself that everything was fine. I had just had an ultrasound a month earlier, and I was able to see the baby's heart beating. It was so amazing!

When I arrived at my doctor's office, his ultrasound machine wasn't working, so he sent me down the street for the ultrasound. He wouldn't reveal any concerns until he had the results. So, off I went to the radiology department just two blocks away, but it felt like I was driving for an eternity.

"Please, God," I wailed as my fists pounded the steering wheel. "Let this baby be okay. I can't lose another one. We already have names picked out. Do you hear me, God! Michael. Gabriel. My child has a name, God. A name. This baby was going to make it!"
I cried and cried between rants because I knew down deep in my heart; something was terribly wrong.

When I arrived, the technician quickly discerned my state of mind and was as pleasant as she could be under the circumstances. She held my hand as she placed the probe on my abdomen and rubbed it all around. I could see the shape of the baby outlined on the screen. I watched as she measured the baby's length. I noticed she was avoiding looking at me, and I knew why. Finally, I broke the silence with the truth that hung like thick, rancid air in the room.

"My baby's heart isn't beating."

The technician looked at me with tears streaming down her face. She didn't need to say anything. As she rubbed the gel from my abdomen, I thanked her and got up from the exam table. Then, I walked, zombie-like, out of the office and into my car. By the time I reached the doctor's office, he had the report. He ushered me into his private office and unceremoniously delivered the news.

"Your baby is dead," he said as if he were providing the weather report.

I didn't think his callousness could get any worse until he said, "We'll have to perform a D&C in case you don't spontaneously abort the entire fetus. In any case, we most likely will have to remove the skull cap."

His insensitive words cut through me like a dull saw blade—each saw tooth cut a new wound in my soul. I stared blankly at him until he broke the silence.

"Are you okay to drive home? Do you want me to call your husband?"

I didn't answer him. Instead, I quickly escaped his stifling office, slamming the door in my wake. I don't know how long I sat bawling in my car, or how long I drove aimlessly, pondering all the questions bouncing in my head like dodge balls. The question balls pummeled me over and over again:

Why did you go swimming? Why didn't you take better care of yourself? they pounded. *Why did you sand that table?*

As I drove on autopilot, I questioned every moment of this pregnancy—just as I had all the times before. I don't know where I went, how long I drove, or even how I found my way back home. All I remember is that the sun had set by the time I willed my numb body to park the car outside of our apartment.

I walked down the cobblestone path leading to my front door, but I didn't want to open the door because I didn't want to face my husband. In my present state of mind, I ranked him right behind the heartless doctor.

How could my husband not even take the day off to be with me? My mind was rattling, even though I had told him to go to work.

I guess I thought I could handle this one just like I had "handled" the others; although, I didn't "handle" any of them. I beat myself up after each miscarriage. It's no wonder I'm not black and blue inside and out. When I finally got up the courage to open the door, Jack was anxiously waiting for me. He had no idea where I was. I could see the worry and concern on his face as his eyes met mine, and I knew that he knew.

The anger I felt toward him dissipated as he took me in his arms and held me. I buried my face on his shoulder, and I drenched his shirt with fresh tears as his embrace offered reassuring comfort. Jack wasn't one to express his emotions, but I knew that on some level, he was feeling this loss too.

Jess was three years old. I had to tell Jess that the baby wasn't going to be born. I explained that the doctor was going to take the baby out early so that he or she could go to heaven. Jess listened intently to what I was telling her. Then, she lifted my blouse, revealing my still swollen belly. I stared at it as it cruelly mocked me.

No baby. Dead baby. Lost baby. Gone baby, gone!

My taunting mind was interrupted by Jess's little voice, "Mommy, can I kiss the baby goodbye?"

If I had to point to a moment that defined this profound loss, it was when my three-year-old curled up next to me on my bed and quietly bent and kissed my belly. Then, she waved "Bye, bye" to our baby.

"Mommy," she smiled, "I saw him fly to heaven."

I believe with all my heart that she did see our baby "fly to heaven." I know that God gave me that moment to help ease the pain. Even now, every nuance of the still-frame moment is etched in my memory: the rumpled bedspread, the flowered curtains fluttering in the breeze, the patch of sun spilling over the bed; it still evokes tears of sadness and loss. Yet, it also gives me great hope that one day I will hold that blessed little soul.

Until then, thank you, God, for carrying me.

Fostering 101

After the miscarriages and before the birth of our beautiful daughter Emily (1991), Jack and I decided to become foster parents. We were foster parents for more than 20 years. We've cared for over 50 children. Jack and I were foster parents for some of the most challenging kids. One of our charges tried to throw himself in the pool every time there was a lightning storm; another ran around the car at breakneck speed every day at parent drop-off at school; another climbed to the top of the monkey bars after school and refused to come down.

One of our caseworkers confessed that they always placed the most difficult cases with us because they knew we could handle them. We couldn't. We were just like any other parents trying to be "experts" at raising children and failing miserably. As the Yiddish saying goes: "He's an expert like a goat's an expert on musicians."

Maybe super-mom status escaped me, but I kept at it. Jack and I even ran a Christian children's home and had thirteen children at one time (another book). We also adopted two children adding to the two of our own. I often tell people I have five children. I count one more child as a member of our family even though she was never adopted—Adilah is our Muslim daughter. Adilah is the reason our family was on Oprah, but I have to spin this yarn a bit longer to tell that part of the story.

The children's home rested (or perhaps it would be more apropos to say "never rested") on five acres and came with kids, a barn, and 4-H horses. I think it's where I discovered that farm living was the life for me. Jack just came along for the ride. Our kids didn't seem too enthralled with farm living either. Emily was the only one who showed any interest in horses, so we got her one. Jessica couldn't care less about farm animals, and our son, Kevin, was much like Jack in his lack of enthusiasm for anything barn related.

The 4-H club met every week in the barn, and I signed Emily and Spit Fire (her paint pony) up right away. Spit Fire was just that—a spitfire. He was untrained and unpredictable. Emily kept with him, though, and her strong will mixed with his fighting spirit. Somehow, they managed to meld.

Emily even showed Spit Fire at the 4-H fair. He was a chubby pony, so we dressed him up like a sumo wrestler, diapers and all. Emily was a skinny little thing riding the sumo wrestler pony in her cowgirl hat and boots. I'm not sure if anyone knew that Spit Fire was a sumo wrestler, but they looked so cute together. I was so proud of my cowgirl daughter. I think there was a part of me living vicariously through Emily.

The mission of the children's home was to keep siblings entering foster care together. So, we often had two to three groups of siblings in addition to our three children: Jessica, Kevin, and Emily. At one time, we had thirteen children—ten from one family. It was a trying time for Jack and me as we tried to juggle all the rigors that accompany children.

Things like teacher conferences, ballet class, and soccer practice/games took up all our time. I remember the time I lost the milk for an entire day. I later discovered it sitting on the floor of the van. Then, there was the time that the toilets were overflowing. Adilah was pushing with all her might on the toilet seat lid screaming, "Oh my gosh. My toilet water is falling out." So many memories! As I said, there are enough memories to fill another book. I finally did write the book, *Melody of my Heartstrings.*

Oprah Lady

Perhaps the most vivid memory I have is of the day that I got "the call." I was in the throes of picking nits out of the heads of eleven children. There was laundry piled literally to the ceiling in the living room, waiting to be washed and dried in the hopes of either drowning or baking any remaining lice. I had a pen in my mouth for some strange reason, and I spit it out when Kevin, holding the phone in my direction, announced, "Oprah is on the phone."

I don't remember my reply, but I'm sure it was snide. I probably said something like, "Yeah, and I'm Queen Elizabeth."

I took the phone and rudely pronounced to "Oprah" that this better be good because I was busy picking lice out of long blonde hair. Have you ever tried to find lice in long blonde hair? It's awful. It's tragic when your bifocals keep slipping off your nose, and you spill your beer all over the floor because you misjudge the distance between your hand and the beer bottle. I wasn't drinking beer, but I was seriously contemplating a secret run to the outside refrigerator in the garage for a quickie when the call came in.

It wasn't Oprah. It was Oprah's assistant. I don't remember her name now, but I had many conversations with the Oprah lady (as she would come to be known in the weeks that followed.) She was calling about Adilah.

Adilah (Adi) came to the children's home from Bangladesh by way of Orlando. She was a beautiful girl who had been horribly disfigured by acid that was thrown in her face. The Oprah show had already done two stories on Adilah's brutal attack and wanted to do a follow-up story about women/girls who are victims of violence. The organization that brought Adi to the United States for a series of surgeries to restore her face gave our name to the show.

"Ok," I managed, "What do you need from me?"

I had no idea those six simple words would turn into a month's worth of back and forth with the Oprah lady at least three days a week. To say these conversations nearly "drove me to drink" is an understatement. They drove me to near insanity. I wondered why I was doing this in the midst of a siege of stubborn lice, which left me no choice but to mayonnaise and bag all the heads in the family. Smother the bastards!

After a while, the lice became part of the background noise of the children's home. Lice, the Oprah lady, teacher conferences, missing milk, soccer practice; all of it became background noise. Isn't that how life is sometimes? Life's just so overwhelming that everything has to be pushed to the background, and you only deal with what is right in front of you at that moment. That's how life got at the children's home. It became one overwhelming day after another.

Somehow, amidst the chaos, I became the writer, videographer, and producer of the Oprah show. I don't know how I got through it, but the Oprah show aired with all of my puzzle pieces fitting into place. It started with my phone voice in the background reading a letter that I wrote about Adilah: "Dear Oprah," (that was the only part left of what I wrote). The Oprah show had edited my letter to the point where I didn't recognize it anymore. Every time the Oprah lady called, I had to read each modified version over the phone to her.

While I was reading in the background, the show flashed to still-frame photos that I took, edited, and emailed to the Oprah show. The segment ended with my home video recording of Adilah riding Emily's horse (also revised, digitized by me, and sent via email).

The whole segment lasted maybe 10 minutes. Oprah never spoke with Adi or me. She would not bring Adi to the studio because the subject matter (violence against women) was somehow too horrible, and Oprah didn't want to scar Adi—as if she weren't already dreadfully scarred.

No one from the Oprah show ever came to our house: no camera crew, no one with a clapboard announcing, "take one," no fancy microphones hanging on a pole. Nothing. To my knowledge, no donation was ever made on Oprah's behalf to the non-profit children's home. After the Oprah show aired, I still shopped at the Harry Chapin Food Bank for food because we couldn't afford a real grocery store on the monthly food budget.

So, our family was featured on Oprah without being featured on Oprah—just background noise. That's all it was. We did receive two oversized tee shirts with the "Oprah Show" logo splattered across the front. I cut one of those tee shirts into rags just the other day. I bet that Oprah doesn't even remember Adilah's story. I guess it was just background noise to her too!

Adi had 26 surgeries while she was with us. When she first joined our family, she was missing one eye, and she had a hole in her face where her nose used to be. She endured tremendous pain during the three years of surgery. I cannot even fathom her anguish. Adi's spirit carried her through everything with an upbeat attitude that defied all odds. We were so blessed to have Adi as part of our family. Adi was such an inspiration to everyone that met her. She inspired me. She inspired all our children. It was only natural that we took Adi with us when we finally left the children's home.

Chapter 29

Unprepared

2001

After the Children's Home

Jack and I had reached the point of exhaustion with 13 children running us ragged. It wasn't just the children that we had to deal with on a regular basis. In addition to the children, we had a constant influx of well-meaning but overpowering volunteers coming and going in the home all day long. There was little to no privacy for anyone in our family.

The woman who was the director of the children's home, Ms. Shelia, was a childless neat-nick with a penchant for spotless tile floors. Our tile floors were white and never spotless. Well, this created a constant source of tension between Ms. Shelia and me. Things reached the breaking point when Ms. Shelia started a daily ritual of inspecting each room in the home.

Jack and I weren't being paid one dime. We were "working" at the children's home for room and board only. Finally, we decided that it was time to focus on *our* kids and ditch the children's home. We only wished to take two of the children in our care with us. At that time, we were caring for another child besides Adilah with medical needs. Her name was Lucy. Lucy was an orphan from Haiti. We asked that Lucy and Adilah accompany our family back to our home when we left the children's home.

Luckily, we had kept our former home and rented it during our tenure at the children's home. That is the home we happily returned to with expectations of privacy, downtime, and my own cleaning schedule. We were so excited until we saw the inside of the house!

I'll never forget the day I entered our old home, and before seeing red, I saw black. That is what our old home was—black. The man who rented it painted almost all the rooms in the house black. On top of that, the pungent smell of his dogs' excrement hit us like a ton of bricks when the door opened. His dogs should have been named "Feces" and "Urine."

We couldn't live in the house until the carpet was torn out, and the house was fumigated and painted. I still have nightmares about it, but we were lucky to have people from our church who assisted in the clean-up, and we moved back in, right before Christmas, December 2001.

We didn't stay long. We still had Emily's horse, which we were paying way too much to board at a rundown barn. The farm bug had bitten me, so we started looking for a small farm. We found our dream home on five acres in 2002 and have been living on the farm ever since. It's like Green Acres reversed: I'm Eddie Albert and Jack's Eva Gabor. We even had a pet pig: Barbie Q. Pig, but she didn't last long because she kept running away, so Jack sent her to live on another farm.

Chapter 30

Unforgivable

The Farm

December 2016

The screaming didn't last long. Both the lobster and Lucy fell into a disturbing silence that did more to unnerve me than the screaming. Although I had planned on sitting in the office to write, I relented and made my way back into the kitchen just to sneak a peek. Lucy was standing over the large boiling pot holding her hand inches from the lid. She looked like a petrified statue—like a freeze-frame from a horror film.

"Just open the lid," I coaxed. "He won't jump out at you. He's dead."

Lucy jumped like I had snuck up behind her and tickled her under her armpits.

"Mom!" She yelled. "Go back to your writing. You're not supposed to be in here. I'm cooking your dinner."

"Okay," I said soothingly. "I was just worried because I didn't hear anything, and I wanted to check on you."

Lucy's eye roll has been perfected over the years. She learned it at the ripe old age of three from Shardé (one of her classmates in preschool). Now, I got the perfect "go away" eye roll from Lucy and quickly retreated to the office to write. So, what if the lobster is overdone and the potatoes aren't boiled correctly? It was still my birthday dinner, and I needed to leave it to Lucy to figure it out for herself.

Back at my keyboard, I reflect that I went outside to search for God. It seems I spend a lot of time searching for Him. Why? I wonder. Am I looking for answers? Of course. How do I know when I find God? How do I know when I find answers? We humans seem to have a fascination with searching for God and answers.

I wonder if ants search for God. What about the donkeys outside my window right now; do they ever comb the pasture for God? I doubt it. I bet they already know that God is with them. He's there, and He's here. I don't have to search for Him, do I? He's been with me since the beginning. God alone has stood by me every step of the way.

I wonder about turmoil because that is what nudges us to reach for God's hand. Turmoil and discontent lead us to search for answers. We search for answers in other people, self-help books, counseling, divorce court, and even Bible study. Searching is a favorite human pastime. That's why the search engine, Google has been such a huge success.

Can I Google God? What would I type? God answers?

I guess I have to know why I'm so intent on finding God in the first place. I think it would be more apropos to say that I'm searching for God's peace. I'm searching for His calm in my storm. When I find His calm and recognize it, I'll thank Him for it. Soon after, I'll get in my car to drive somewhere and end up cursing out the driver that just cut me off. Or, I'll get to the school to pick up Lucy, and she'll give me a perfected eye roll, and I'll want to smack her for her lack of gratitude that I remembered to pick her up from school.

Every Sunday in church, the Catholics say, "Peace be with you." Then, in the parking lot after church, they all beep at one another and block each other from leaving their parking spaces.

Peace is fleeting. It'll fleet right in us and right out of us before we even know it's there. So how do we keep it? Isn't that the age-old question? How do we keep God alone at the helm? If we could learn to do that, then I believe we'd all be at peace, and there'd be no need for Yiddish curses. But the sad truth is that we all give the devil his due. As the Yiddish would say: "If you give the devil a hair, he'll want the whole beard!"

Jessica is the reason that I went to the pasture. She's the reason that I asked God to show up. She's the reason that my heart and soul are so broken right now. It's her daily struggle that makes me cry out to God because I cannot bear to see my child going through this.

Isn't life a beautiful struggle? Aren't our struggles what define us? I Googled struggle quotes to see if I could find some wisdom about struggles. This Mahatma Gandhi quote came up.

"Your beliefs become your thoughts, Your thoughts become your words, Your words become your actions, Your actions become your habits, Your habits become your values, Your values become your destiny."

We all struggle every day. It's what we do with our struggles that matter. What do our beliefs, words, thoughts, and actions say about us? What will be written in our obituary? A guy named Leslie recently died, and his obituary was Googled thousands of times because of its offensiveness. I Googled Leslie's obituary: "...at a young age, Leslie quickly became a model example of bad parenting...Leslie's passing proves that evil does, in fact, die...." It went on, but it's pretty clear that Leslie isn't going to be missed, and his legacy is less than stellar.

Speaking of less than stellar legacies, I could write an excellent tribute for Aaron. I'd probably add a few Yiddish curses as well. Somehow, I'd tie in this one: "If he were twice as smart, he'd be an idiot!" And maybe this one: "When a man is too good for the world, he's bad for his wife (in this case ex-wife)." And for Aaron and his girlfriend: "They are both in love, he with himself and she with herself." I'd have to change the wording a bit, but I'm confident that I could top Leslie's obituary Google hits with little difficulty.

I wonder if God would approve of my legacy. If God were going to write my obituary, what would He say? Good and faithful servant? A woman after My own heart? I don't think He would approve of my desire to destroy Aaron. God probably wants me to forgive Aaron. Really. Forgiveness requires tremendous strength of character. Forgiveness means that I cannot cast Yiddish curses on Aaron anymore. Forgiveness means that I have to admit that I am a flawed human being, and I do not possess the ability to cast the anger aside to make room for forgiveness.

"Dinner's ready!"

Lucy's announcement interrupted my forgiveness thoughts.

"I'll revisit this later," I say aloud as if speaking these words will somehow make my heart and mind stand up and take notice. I stand up and proclaim to God that I'll think about forgiving the man that hurt my child.

Shortly after my pronouncement, I see Jess being wheeled to the dinner table by her sister, Emily. *Who am I kidding? She is my kid. No one messes with my kid!* That's what my heart was screaming as I walked to the dining room and saw my family gathered around one giant red lobster in the middle of the table. Just one. That's all we could afford on Jack's teaching salary. The rest of the family was getting shrimp. The giant lobster was mine alone—the birthday girl!

"Happy birthday to you!" They were all singing as I took my place at the head of the table. I lose myself in the moment, surrounded by my loving family, singing beautifully off-key. I allow myself to feel at peace. I might even allow a sliver of forgiveness to inch into my soul. Will the shred of forgiveness stay? I wonder as I crack the lobster's tail off with savage vivacity.

Chapter 31

Untangled

February 2017

Three months have passed since the birthday dinner. Over these three months, I have frequented the forgiveness reflection pool over and over again. I even committed these verses to memory: "Put on therefore...a heart of compassion...and forgiving each other...even as the Lord forgave you..." (Col. 3:12-13)

I have to repeat this Bible verse regularly, especially when I wrestle with myself in the muck and mire of UN. That one little syllable keeps popping up in my forgiveness battle. Unforgiveness (I know this is not a word, but it fits) rears its ugly head every time I read a new motion from Jessica's attorney concerning the "reckless dissipation of marital money."

The Land of UN is where I spend my time when I hear my little granddaughter yell to her mother, "I'm not supposed to tell you that I went to Disney World with Daddy and Miss Dolores." At those times, UN seems like a perfect place for me—Drama Momma in the Land of UN.

What kind of UN are we talking about here?

It's the kind of UN that rots you from the inside out. It's the kind of UN that makes your frown lines become permanent crevices in your face. It's UNthinkable. It's UNrelenting. It's UNsafe. It's the kind of UN that doesn't destroy the one it is aimed at, no it's the UN that destroys the one who harbors it.

This UN will destroy me if I don't wake up, look up, stand up, and dress up in God's armor to fight it. I know I cannot do this alone. I can't leave UN behind if I'm not willing to name it, face it, and destroy it once and for all.

The other day, I gave Jessica a pair of pink boxing gloves to hang on the back of her wheelchair. Maybe I could use those boxing gloves in the Land of UN? The gloves are labeled, "fighting pretty." There's nothing pretty in the Land of UN. I can't wear those gloves there.

Fighting pretty—what an oxymoron. Is there anything pretty about fighting? Is there such a thing as a beautiful battle? I think so. Jessica is fighting pretty, especially when she is in the land of Tampa General Hospital.

Tampa General has become our home away from home. Jessica and I make the two and a half hour trek three days a week. At the hospital, Jessica fights pretty through three hours of therapy: physical, occupational, and cognitive. Her stamina and determination shine through as she rides the bike to exercise her nearly paralyzed left leg, lifts her affected left arm, and writes down facts to help her with recall. She fights pretty with her beautiful smile and an amazingly positive attitude. Jessica takes fighting pretty to a whole new level!

I don't fight pretty. I just fight. Sometimes, instead of fighting, I write. Writing is my fight. Writing is my way of sorting things out. The keyboard and the computer are my boxing ring. Sometimes I write to stay sane. Sometimes I write to stay focused.

Often, I write because it is how I talk to God. When I write, I fight my inner battle—like a chess match with my conscience. I don't want the devil to declare checkmate with my temper. I want to win this battle, but I wouldn't be honest if I didn't say it is a daily battle, and the score is probably tied right now.

When I started to spin this yarn, it was my birthday. I was celebrating 58 years on this earth. My chest pains have subsided since I started writing. I think the pains were due to Nana jarring—Nana jumping on the trampoline with a very active four-year-old. In any case, I got my heart checked and, although it's taken a licking, it's still ticking.

Chapter 32

UNderestimated

Lucy

I've been writing this story since my birthday. Now, it is almost Jessica's birthday. Lucy had a birthday over these past months too. She's seventeen now, hard to believe. Lucy was only 16-months-old when she came to live with us. We called her our "hallelujah baby" because the only word she knew was hallelujah, and she'd yell it over and over again to get a reaction out of the other kids at the children's home. Every morning, Lucy would throw her arms over her head and yell hallelujah to announce she was awake.

Lucy learned hallelujah in the orphanage in Haiti. In the orphanage, they yelled hallelujah every time they received food, blankets, bottles, or diapers. You name it; they shouted hallelujah. I remember how adorable Lucy was when she arrived on our doorstep one day. I was expecting her, but perhaps I wasn't expecting her to show up the way she did.

Two people a (woman and a man) were standing on the porch when I opened the door. Between them was a car seat holding a sleeping baby in a blue dress and black patent leather shoes.

"Hello," they said in unison. "Here, she is." They started to leave before I could ask their names or invite them in. I didn't even have a chance to say thank you before they had turned and started back to the car.

"Wait!" I yelled frantically. "Where's her stuff? Did she come with instructions? What's her name?"

The woman started back towards me. "She was handed to me from the lady on the airplane. That woman did not speak English. She didn't have anything with her except the bottle which is in the car seat. We had to buy a car seat. We didn't get any paperwork or a diaper bag or anything. We had instructions to pick up a baby and to bring her to the host family.

We had to call to get your address after we got her. They failed to tell us your house would be two and a half hours away from the airport," she said. "Oh, one more thing." The woman looked at me with a mixture of pity and a hint of anger (I guess it was due to the two and a half-hour drive). "I think her name is Pat because the lady from the plane kept pointing to her and saying 'Pat.'"

"Thank you," I said. "Would you like to come in and at least have something to eat or drink?"

"No," the woman replied. "We have a long ride back. She'll probably need to be changed when she wakes up. You can keep the car seat." Then, she made a hasty retreat to the car, and the two of them were gone, leaving me alone with a sleeping child on my doorstep.

"Well, hello, Pat," I said to the sleeping baby as I carried her into the house. "Welcome home."

The house was quiet. Jack had taken the kids to a 5K walk for cancer. I was supposed to go to the walk too, but I had to wait for Pat's arrival, and then I was going to meet them with our new charge. Instead of loading Pat into the car, I called the director of Healing Hands, the organization that sent Pat to our doorstep.

"Tina," I said as I looked at the sleeping baby, "I received a little package today, but it seems the package was missing some instructions and other important necessities like a passport or something indicating her name. I was told her name is Pat."

"Pat?" Tina asked. "Who's Pat?"

I told her about the new arrival.

"You mean Palucy!" Tina exclaimed. "She wasn't supposed to be there for another week. What happened?"

"I don't know," I said. "Jack received a call from the people at the orphanage earlier today. They said that we should expect the child to be here by early evening." I sighed. "You know how men are," I said. "They're not big on details."

"Well," Tina said, "that's a surprise."

"Is her name 'Palucy?'" I asked puzzled. "Because the lady seemed to think that they called her 'Pat' at the orphanage."

"I don't know," Tina replied. "We haven't even received her paperwork yet."

"Well, I'm not calling her Palucy," I said. "Maybe we'll just shorten it to 'Lucy' until we find out her real name."

My next call was to the director of the orphanage. She didn't answer, and I didn't know what to call my newest addition to the children's home. So, I made an executive decision that Palucy was now Lucy, and Pat was no longer.

It wasn't long before the sleeping angel in the car seat was the wide-awake, newly named Lucy. I changed the squirming bundle of joy and then decided that she must be hungry, but I didn't have a clue how to feed this adorable child.

Lucy didn't have an upper lip, but that just added to her cuteness in my eyes. Where her lip should have been, she had two little teeth between two gaping holes on either side.

"How do I feed you?" I asked Lucy as if she'd tell me. "What do I feed you?"

I found some baby food in the pantry and fixed a lovely plate of ground lamb and mashed peas. I put the food in Lucy's mouth, and it came right out of her nose! Lucy laughed. I laughed. I wasn't sure what to do next, but Lucy solved the problem for me. She put her finger in the hole in her lip and pushed the food down somehow. I'm not even sure how she did it, but she managed to feed herself with this method.

The bottle had the top cut off so that it did not require sucking. Lucy took it from me and showed me how she positioned it just so in one of the holes in her lip. She drank her bottle with gusto. I was amazed at her ability to adapt and her sweet disposition. She didn't cry. She didn't even seem distressed by her new surroundings. She looked right at home already.

After the feeding, I loaded Lucy back in her car seat and took her to meet her new daddy and all her brothers and sisters at the cancer walk. It was love at first sight. I don't think Lucy's feet touched the floor at all that day. Everyone wanted to hold her and play with her. She willingly went from outstretched arms to outstretched arms soaking in all the attention.

When Adi took Lucy in her arms, I expected that Lucy might cry because of Adi's scarred face (it's a little scary at first glance). No, Lucy didn't cry. Lucy squealed with delight at being held in another set of arms. After thinking about it, it occurred to me that Lucy probably was not held much at all in the orphanage. I know she had a crib-mate, and the two of them played together in their crib much of the day. I wondered how often the understaffed and overworked orphanage volunteers were able to give one-on-one attention to their small charges.

There is one lesson, I prayed my children would take away from the children's home, and it was that they would be accepting of everyone despite their outward appearance. I could tell by the way that my children held and cuddled with Lucy that she would fit right in with the family. Not one of my kids balked at holding or cuddling with this child that had two holes in her face where her lip should have been.

Lucy fit right in with our family as if she had always been a part of the children's home landscape. She didn't walk when she first arrived, but that didn't last long.

I think the children's home was the antithesis of the orphanage. In the orphanage, Lucy was lucky to be taken out of her crib and held a few times a day. At the children's home, Lucy was lucky to be put in her crib for a nap once a day. Lucy's entire waking moments were filled with stimulation from all nine children.

Tony and Julie were in charge of dancing and singing. Jess, Emily, and Adilah were in charge of making Lucy laugh, blow kisses, and talk. Kevin saw to it that Lucy practiced walking. Leandra, Shelia, and Joe made sure that Lucy said hallelujah over and over again. The child never lacked attention, and she reveled in it. By the time Lucy was three, she had scored in the "superior" range in all areas of development, except for speech, which was due to her cleft lip and palate.

Over the next few months at the children's home, Lucy underwent several surgeries to correct her cleft lip and palate. It was a trying time for our family because Adi was undergoing surgeries too. I still don't know how Jack and I did it. We had lots of help from friends and family and were able to get through it somehow, but the strain took its toll, and we soon came to the realization that it was time to go back home.

We knew that we'd continue to care for Lucy and Adi, though, and we eventually adopted Lucy. It took us many years to go through the adoption process; she was seven years old when the judge finally signed the adoption papers.

The early years were not easy for Lucy. She had to undergo many additional surgeries and still, at the age of 17, has one more operation to go. Over the years, we finally got Lucy's paperwork from Haiti and found out her real name, Esther. To everyone else that meets her, she is Esther, but to us, she will always be Lucy.

Chapter 33

UNwanted

Kevin

This is my son's story. It is the one that I have struggled most with writing because I have trouble conveying the emotion that embodies it, but I'm going to do my best to portray his story as honestly as I can.

Picture, if you will, never having a home to call your own, never knowing from one day to the next where you will be or who you will be living with. Now, imagine that you are only a child, and your fate rests in the hands of adults who are strangers that float in and out of your life. These adults tell you that it is their job to protect you, and you have to trust them. You want to believe these strangers because they are all you have standing between you and an abusive mother.

You and your brother have been taken away from her several times already, but you are too little to remember. Your first real memory is when you were about five, and one of the strangers showed up at your mother's doorstep, and you remember your mother crying. The stranger tells you to pack your things.

You don't know what to do. You're not supposed to talk to strangers or get in strangers' cars. This person tells you that she is taking you away to protect you. You want to leave, but your mother needs you, doesn't she? All sorts of emotions are running through your brain as the stranger hustles you into your room. You want to cry, but you have to be brave for your little brother. He's only three, and he is crying. You hug him and tell him you will never leave him.

What do you pack? You have to pack for him too. The stranger tries to help you, but she doesn't know what is important to you. She just wants you to take some clothes. She tells you that there will be toys for you at your new home. You believe her. You throw a few clothes in a garbage bag (and sneak some favorite toys in as well), grab your brother's hand and follow the stranger to the car.

You only look back once and see your mother sitting on the couch, crying. You picture her in broken pieces. That memory is etched in your brain as you gaze through the back window of the car at your house, fading in the distance.

The caseworker takes you to the home of new strangers, and after about an hour, leaves you there. She says she'll be back to see you soon. These strangers are supposed to be like parents and care for you in their home. At first, you and your brother don't talk to these new people. You stay in the nice room they give you and play with the cool toys. Soon, you start to like this new place and these "parents" who take you to church and the movies.

After a few months, you start to hope that the caseworker will let you and your brother stay here. You even allow a glimmer of hope to tickle the back of your brain: Maybe they'll adopt us. Sometimes, when you lie in your comfy bed at night, you allow yourself to dream that this will be your forever home and that you and your brother will be loved forever by these parents.

Then, it happens—your hope is shattered because the caseworker, who promised to protect you, comes back into your life and tells you that you are going back to your mother.

Now, most children would be happy to return to their mothers. However, you are not like most children because your mother doesn't bring you cookies and milk or tuck you in at night. Instead, you never have enough to eat, and sometimes you don't have a bed to sleep in. Sometimes, you have to tuck Mommy into bed because she is sick. Mommy also brings very mean men into your life. Yet, you have no say in what happens to you because the lady who is supposed to protect you tells you that your mother is better now.

You wonder, what does better mean? Is she going to stop putting that needle in her arm that makes her sick? Is she going to buy food and bake brownies? You don't know what it means. All you know is that you and your brother have to throw all your stuff into the garbage bags again and say goodbye to the nice foster mom who did bake brownies and the foster dad who played ball with you. This time, you cry as you take your brother's hand and follow the caseworker to her car. As you leave, you tell yourself that you will never hope again.

So, you return to your mother, and you quickly learn that she is not better. She's still doing drugs and leaving you alone to fend off the boogeymen she's brought back into your life. You, being the older brother, know that it is your job to protect your little brother from these men that hurt you and your little brother in ways you never want to remember.

Sometimes, you can't defend him, and you cry yourself to sleep at night.

Then, a new caseworker comes into your life and tells you that you are leaving your mother again. And so, it goes, you and your little brother grab your garbage bags full of clothes and a few treasured toys, and you leave to go to someone else's house. Someone you don't know. You are scared. No, you are terrified. You are terrified that these people might be mean, or worse—you might grow to love them and then be taken away again. For two years, this is the roller coaster life you and your brother live, and you hate it. You learn never to trust what these adults tell you, and you vow never to let yourself hope.

Fast forward to our home. Kevin was eight when he and his brother Joe walked into our lives with their garbage bags full of memories better left forgotten. They were covered with bug bites, dirty and scared.

They had been placed in at least eight homes in the six years that they were in foster care. When they came to us, I wanted more than anything to give them both the love and support of a forever home.

We grew to love both boys as they became a part of our family. We knew that they would most likely be put up for adoption because the courts finally decided that it was time to sever the mother's parental rights. We planned to adopt both of them. Then, something went dreadfully wrong.

I've never written about the painful decision that we had to make after the boys entered our lives. This decision deeply affected our entire family, and most of all, had a profound impact on Kevin and his brother, Joe. It was a decision that haunts me every day, but I still believe it was the right decision at the time.

In short, we had to reevaluate our decision to adopt both Kevin and Joe. Both boys had suffered so many tragedies in their young lives. Joe was left deeply scarred and needed specialized help. Sadly, after many consultations with doctors and therapists, we determined that Joe would be better served in a therapeutic setting where he could get the support he so desperately needed. We would still see him, but we did not feel we would be the best family to adopt him.

Like I said, to this day, I struggle with the decision to adopt Kevin and not Joe. I know in my heart that it was the right decision, but it still haunts me. It haunts me mostly because I know that Kevin made a promise to his brother that he would never leave him. I cannot imagine the burden this put on Kevin's heart. I cannot describe the pain that he must have felt when Joe left.

We loved Joe. We truly did. We simply could not keep him in our home, and we wanted to give Kevin at least a chance to have a family to call his own. Foster parenting is so hard when you know that these broken children are yearning for a family, yet most of them just float in and out of your home because they are frequently reunited with their biological parents time and time again.

When they are finally put up for adoption, the years of turmoil have made them angry, despondent, and fearful. Sometimes, the system has failed a child to the point of irreparable damage. That is what we feared happened to Joe, yet we saw a glimmer of hope for Kevin, so we made the decision to try to save Kevin.

Kevin has had his share of rough patches since his adoption. For a while, he drifted in and out of our lives. I knew he was angry, hurt, and confused and would have to find his *own* way in life. I never stopped loving him. I never stopped believing in him. I never stopped knowing that he was and always would be my son.

When he was sixteen, he left our home in search of his "real family" (he had two sisters and a brother who had been taken away from his mother years before he and Joe were put into foster care). We let him go because we had to. He would never be a part of our family until he wrestled with the demons of his past. I believed in my heart that he would come back. I believed that he would realize that we were and always would be his forever family. I believed that he would one day know that we never stopped loving him.

For four years, I waited to see my son.

It was my birthday, and we went out to eat. I was sitting at the table when a tall, handsome young man came over to join us. At first, I wasn't sure that I was indeed seeing what I thought I was seeing, but Kevin came over and hugged me and said, "Hello Mama!" He always called me Mama. I put my arms around him and held on tight because I never wanted to lose him again. My tears drenched his shirt, but I didn't care. My son was back—that was the best birthday present I could have ever received.

I looked at this young man standing in front of me, and I thanked God that He sent him back into my life. I missed him so much. I almost lost hope that he would return to our family. I thought that he never believed he was loved as deeply as all our children. I worried that he just didn't feel like he belonged to us.

Then, Kevin gave me my birthday present, and I knew that I was wrong. My birthday present was a picture Kevin had framed. It was a crude pencil drawing I had made for him when he and his brother first came to live with us. I remember drawing the picture (I have never been even remotely artistically inclined, and this picture was no exception).

I can still picture Kevin, Joe, and I sitting on the couch laughing about how silly my drawing was. The stick people in our family were almost as big as our house. Our car was smaller than the people, and our bird was bigger than the cats, but that didn't matter. What mattered to Kevin was that he and his brother were finally in a family portrait. They belonged in this picture just as much as everyone else.

After Kevin handed me the picture, he gave me a laminated letter tied with a bow. He took such care in these gifts. It made me cry even harder. Here is the letter:

Mom,

Twelve years ago, I was a scared, lost, and confused little boy. Nowhere to run, nowhere to find a safe place, and no one to show me the meaning of love. When I was eight, you accepted me in, and I felt that you not only accepted me in your heart but into your family. When you first drew a picture with me, your little boy in the picture, you made me realize how important I was to you and everyone else.

When I look back twelve years ago, I see a boy who struggled with obstacles in his life, but you always were there to put me back on my feet because I was your son. I know I have made mistakes, but you were always there pushing me in the right way and never letting me forget how much you and the rest of the family loved me. You made me realize what true love and lasting love was between a family.

I just want you to know how much I appreciate everything you have done for me and provided in my life: a family, a true mom, and a safe place to run to when I was scared and confused. Mom, I love you so much, and I wanted to give you a gift that means as much to you as it does to me.

Love,
Your son, Kevin

Reflection

Kevin passed away from a drug overdose three years after I started writing this book. Since then, I met with the First Lady at the White House to discuss opioid addiction. Today, my heart still breaks for my son. All I can hope for is knowing he is finally at peace.

Chapter 34

UNspeakable

Early Years

When I look at my broken children: Kevin, Lucy, and Adi, I can't help but think about my broken childhood. My scars were not visible from the outside, but they were festering on the inside for years. I was a shy, aloof child in school. At home, I stayed in my room and read Nancy Drew and Hardy Boys books. I had the misfortune of being left-handed and attending Catholic School in the '60s. Nuns back then believed in conformity. I was forced to conform to the rest of my right-handed classmates.

I have no good memories of my early school days—not one. I do remember being regularly hit with a ruler on my left hand every time I picked up a crayon or pencil. I remember not being allowed to march in the Easter Parade in first grade because I had to sit at the piano (the kind with the tall back) and practice writing my name with my right hand. As an added punishment, the nun placed my Easter bonnet on the top of the piano to remind me what I was missing because I was too stupid to use my correct hand.

Stupid was a word that played like a broken record in my head—stupid, stupid, stupid. Every morning, I got up feeling stupid, and every night I went to bed feeling stupider because I couldn't complete my homework with my right hand. My step-mother, Dotty, was a conformity freak too. Dotty continued the nun's evil methods with me—all that was missing was the habit.

I learned to write with my right hand eventually (probably by third grade), but not before the damage was already done. I was labeled stupid and dumb, and I became the brunt of the school bully's jokes and harassment. One time, in eighth grade, the nun stepped out of the room, and the class bully came up behind me and slapped me out of my chair. Everyone laughed.

I got unsteadily to my feet, still hearing ringing in my head. I didn't hear the laughter as much as I saw it on everyone's face. I felt like I was removed from the room at that moment. I didn't want to stay. I sat back in my seat and cried silently in my folded arms on my desk.

"Gwen!" I heard the nun's shrill voice through my ringing ears. "Why are you crying?"

I didn't answer her. I left the room then. Not physically. I floated away. My body stayed behind to take whatever abuse the nun was dishing out, but my mind left. I went down the hall and watched a kid come out of one of the classrooms on crutches with someone following, holding her books.

Back in my classroom, I think the nun was still scolding me for crying, and the kids were all still laughing. Thankfully, there wasn't much time left before class was dismissed.

The bell rang, and we were excused. I didn't wait around to find out what my punishment would be for crying in class. I practically ran out of the room to the hallway, where I had "seen" the kid on crutches. There she was. She and her book carrier were leading the pack of kids switching classes. I was amazed and confused. That was the first time I "floated away" from the scene of abuse but certainly not the last.

I became very adept at leaving the scene of abuse. I had lots of opportunities at school and home. Floating (as I called it) saved me on many occasions. It saved me from playground hell, and it lessened some terrible experiences at home that I really cannot remember now.

That's the thing about survival; the human mind is capable of enduring so much trauma because it provides us with ways to adapt and cope. I adapted and coped as best I could as a child.

One of my coping mechanisms was running. I was exceedingly fast. I discovered this running ability when we lived in a neighborhood with tons of kids who loved to race one another. I joined in the races and soon won all of them. It got to be a joke in our neighborhood that no one could beat me in a race even if I were barefoot. So, I raced barefoot. I still won. Then, the fathers in the neighborhood would challenge me to a race, and I'd beat them too—barefoot.

At school, I was the stupid kid with no friends. At home, I became the fastest kid in the neighborhood whom no one could beat. It was the first time I felt like I was somebody. Naturally, when the county eighth-grade track meet was posted in our school, I signed up. I didn't know how I was going to get there, but I was going to run in that race by God! There were only two girls who signed up, but the school had no say as to whether or not we went, they just told us to get there on our own.

My parents gave in and brought me to the track meet. I'm guessing it was because I was running for the Catholic school, and they didn't want to look bad in front of the nuns and priests. My parents were not big on supporting anything we did as kids. This was the only time I ever saw Dotty at a track meet. My father did attend one other meet years later when I was competing at the state level in high school.

It was pitiful watching me and one other girl prepare for the 4x4 relay. Only two teams were competing in this race: Catholic school vs. Catholic school. Typically, you'd have four runners for a 4x4 relay. Since we only had two, we each positioned ourselves at the halfway point on the track. I was the second runner. The gun sounded, and our first runner made a valiant attempt to keep up with her competitor. She fell behind.

By the time the other team's first runner handed off the baton to the second runner, our girl had not even turned the first corner. It looked hopeless. I got the baton well after the runner next to me had taken off and was about to pass the baton to their anchor. I didn't just start running; I blasted off like a rocket. I sprinted like never before. I felt like my feet were on fire even though they had shoes on them for once. As I ran, I heard the announcer suddenly come alive with excitement.

"Would you look at that!" he yelled. "I think she's going to catch that girl."

The people in the stands were standing and clapping as I rounded the bend and saw the third girl just ahead of me handing the baton to girl number four. I picked up the pace. The announcer was saying something about this being the fastest 220-yard time they've ever witnessed at this meet.

I remember glancing at the stands where my parents were to see if they, too, were standing and cheering. Big mistake. I faltered. I didn't fall, but I slowed just enough that I knew I wasn't going to catch girl number four. I don't remember seeing my parents.

After the race, many people came up to me and commented about my exceptional speed. One man told me that my time beat the high school state record. Later, in the long jump, my 14' 8" jump tied the county high school record. I wasn't able to run the 100-yard dash because I false started twice. Otherwise, I was told that I would have won the all-around trophy, but I didn't care. After all these years of being the stupid Catholic school dummy, I was now a somebody.

The next day, the eighth grade was abuzz with the news. "Did you hear about Gwen?" The shock was evident in their voices. "She ran really fast, and she won the long jump!"

Some kids and even some nuns congratulated me. Being somebody in Catholic school lasted the rest of my eighth-grade year (about two months). No one picked on me anymore. I don't know if it was because of my track star status or because of my one and only friend, Maryanne.

Maryanne was another outcast who smelled like a farm (probably because she lived on a farm) and was at least a foot taller than the tallest kid in our class. She was a good friend to have around when someone wanted to pick a fight. Maryanne was great at making herself appear even bigger than she was. No one messed with Maryanne, and through osmosis, no one messed with me.

Somehow, I graduated eighth grade despite my abysmal grades. I think my GPA might have been a 1.0. I was the kid that was passed on to the next grade because no one wanted me in their classroom for more than one year. I went on to public high school, where I joined the track team and got involved as a classroom assistant with special education kids. I was a new person in high school. No one knew me because most of the kids from Catholic grade school went to Catholic high school. That was just fine with me.

The new me was a straight "A" student. The new me was popular but still shy. The new me stood up to bullies of all kinds, especially the ones that picked on my special ed kids. I was also published in high school. The school news carried an article I wrote about my special ed kids. It was written from my heart, and I got high praise from all my teachers for my excellent insight. I didn't tell anyone that my insight came from personal experience during my elementary years.

High school is when I decided that I would be a special education teacher because I could relate to those kids. I knew what it was like to be singled out because something about the way you learned, the way you looked, or the way you acted was different.

I'm proud to say that I never wallowed in self-pity during my growing up years. God knows—and he does—that I had ample opportunity for wallowing. I could have joined the pigs in my old farm neighborhood. I could have remained stuck in the mud, but wallowing was not an option for me. Instead, I persevered. I prayed a lot and asked God to direct my path.

Knowing what it was like to be sad and lonely, I became an advocate for kids who I thought might be sad and lonely too. Even at the age of eight, I was well aware of the plight of less fortunate kids. Instead of wallowing, I decided to help Jerry's kids. Every year during the weekend of the Jerry Lewis Telethon, my sister and I organized a "carnival" in my back yard. Again, I don't know where my parents were, but we were able to enlist the help of our other siblings and some neighborhood kids, and we always had a great event.

One year, I put my little sister in a box and told her she was the candy machine. People put money in a hole in the box, and she'd hand out a candy bar through another hole in the box. Never mind that it was over 80 degrees outside (who knows what it was inside the box), and all the candy was melting. The candy machine was a big hit and raised tons of money.

After the event, my sister and I would load up our radio flyer wagon with jars of change and walk downtown to the Jerry Lewis telethon office (yes, there was an office). They probably put the office there just for us! We'd hand the lady behind the desk all our jars of change from the carnival, wave, and say, "See you next year."

We never knew how much money we raised. We never hung around to get our jars back or to watch the lady count the change. I just know that God must have been smiling at our naive trust that we were saving many of Jerry's kids with our pitiful yearly donation. Somehow, I think God found a way to multiply the gift. I knew in my heart that it wasn't the amount that mattered; it was the fact that we gave it from our hearts that mattered to God and Jerry's kids.

Reflection

Now, looking back, I thank God that He gave me such a giving spirit. I thank Him that He allowed the trials into my life that shaped me. I know that trials can either destroy us or make us stronger. I am thankful that my ordeals gave me the strength to endure and overcome. My life has not been easy, but then whose life is?

Chapter 35

UNcomfortable

February 2017

Last night I went to my Bible study. We're learning about not so easy lives. One of the things that came up was the fact that God puts His people in situations that are less than comfortable. Uncomfortable is a common theme throughout the lives of Biblical characters. It's uncanny how many of God's chosen people spent time in the Land of UN. David was in the midst of untold conflict, strife, and battles. Job had unfathomable misfortune but never lost faith in God. Mary was unmarried and pregnant. The list of Biblical characters with terrible burdens is endless.

The natural question we all ask is, "Why does God allow this strife into the lives of His people?"

I ask that. I ask it over and over again. "Why, God?" becomes my constant refrain.

"Why did you allow my mother to die? Why did you let me be punished for being left-handed? Why did I have to float away from so many situations? Why did my father marry a woman who didn't know how to be a mother to me? Why did you allow me to drink myself into oblivion..." Okay, maybe that one was my own free will.

I've asked God why on so many occasions, but perhaps the most distressing "why" of all came today when I stood in the barn alone and cried my heart out over my daughter, Jessica. Today, God had finally gotten my complete attention, and it only took him 58 years to get me to my breaking point!

Perhaps it was last night's Bible study. Who am I kidding? It was last night's Bible study that brought me to this point. It's grief beyond any grief I've ever felt. I've felt grief for myself. I've felt grief for others' misfortune. I've felt grief for Adi and Lucy, but none so strongly as I have for Jessica.

Despair and misery are not feelings I wish to birth. Mourning is not a place I want to be. It's not where I want to stay. I have to confront it and allow the sorrow to come out before it takes root. No one can explain what it is like to cry out to God alone. It's the most solitary experience anyone can have. So, I will not try and describe it. I just know that there is something about tears that wash one's soul. I suppose God could have designed us differently, but "washing" is so symbolic, as is salt. I believe it is why our tears are salty.

The Bible tells us that we are to be "the salt of the earth." I wonder if any of us could be God's salt if we didn't first salt ourselves with an honest cry? I'm not talking about a surface cry. I'm talking about a gut-wrenching, from the heart and soul cry that is only for God alone to hear and see. That's what cleanses us, a desperate cry for help that only God can answer. Until then, we cannot be salt because we haven't been salted ourselves. That's what I think. I think God only used salted people. His people were ordinary enough, but they all had one thing in common—they were all salted.

There is one thing I learned in Bible study; strife is the only thing that brings us closer to God. We don't seem to seek Him in daily life, mundane moments. We look for God when things are rough, times are tough. It seems that the Bible characters that encountered the most strife turned out to be the ones that God relied on the most. There was nothing extraordinary about any of them, yet they became God's heroes. I want to be God's hero because there's nothing extraordinary about me.

So, I asked God how I can be his salt. I know God doesn't answer aloud anymore, but he does put a yearning in us through the Holy Spirit. My longing is to write. I'm compelled to do it. It helps me, and I want it to help others. I want to salt the earth with my writing. I asked the Holy Spirit to guide the rest of my words. I asked God to send them wherever they should go.

After I asked the Holy Spirit to guide my writing, I immediately started wrestling with the Yiddish cursing side of my brain. It didn't take long for the Aaron curses to sneak into my head, especially after I received a particularly nasty text from him. Instead, I prayed, "God be with him." I figured that is all I can muster right now.

"God be with him," I said even though I'm not sure I meant it. I'm still trying to fake it until I make it.

Chapter 36

UNchained

The Divorce

The particularly nasty text I received was telling me that he (Aaron) is sick of me "running to the lawyer every time I need something from him."

"Me!" I'm not the one divorcing him. Why do I get texts from Aaron when he is divorcing Jess?

He went on, "It must be nice to have unlimited money to spend to have your lawyer write emails..."

It's not *my* lawyer. She is Jess's lawyer, and Jess hired her to do just that—communicate on Jess's behalf.

Aaron then told me that he gave Jessica $11,000 when he dropped her off at our house and accused me of only caring about the money.

Of course, I got sucked right into the dialog and immediately forgot about my four-word prayer, "God be with him." I allowed Aaron to shop vac me right into his crazy mixed-up world. I let my tornado temper spin us faster and faster into texting madness. Then, I realized what I was doing. I stopped.

I texted him, "This is not my divorce. I am not allowing you to steal my peace anymore, and I'm not giving it to you either. From now on, you will only hear from Jessica's lawyer. God be with you."

He texted back, "I was encouraged by my attorney to reach out to you guys to try and solve this amicably and without the attorneys for certain things. This makes the process quicker and also doesn't cost us any money.

If you still feel you don't want to have contact with me, then so be it."

So be it, Aaron. I didn't text. Then I whispered this silent prayer that I didn't feel in my heart: "God be with him."

I cannot spin this yarn without relating the divorce story. I tell it because it is such an integral part of what has happened to Jessica and our family. To not tell it would be like leaving a gaping pot-hole in the middle of a road. I can't go around it. I must tell it, but I must try to relate it with honesty and compassion.

Honesty is pretty straightforward. I can be brutally honest about the way this is going. Compassion is a different story. Compassion means that I must examine my motives and use my words carefully. I might even have to refrain from Aaron bashing and Bulldog Anne and Sponge Steve bashing. Humor works. I like humor—especially the biting kind.

It's not easy using humor to describe a bitter divorce, of which I've become an integral part. I feel like I'm a "party" to this divorce that I never asked for and never in a million years thought I would be joining. This is no party.

Aaron's "amicable" agreement includes such wording as "parties would agree to waive any and all claims regarding dissipation, waste, etc." It goes on to say "including, but not limited to, the donation money that the family received as a result of the wife's unfortunate health issue that has resulted in her disability."

That's funny. The donation money was collected for Jess's medical fund, as advertised. It wasn't for the family, and Aaron wasted it on frivolous trips and expensive exercise equipment while his wife was in a rehabilitation hospital five hours north fighting for her life. Despite repeated requests from Jess's attorney, Aaron produced scant evidence showing how much money was spent on Jessica's medical needs.

In all, Aaron received over $30,000. During the time that Jess was at Anne's house, she became an expert on all things HGTV. Aaron (or his mom) would park her in front of the TV in the morning. She'd still be there in the evening when Eva came home. I'd know this because Eva would tell me.

It was a rare occasion when a member of Jess's family was permitted to visit her. I was there twice and, both times, Jess was in her chair watching HGTV. Aaron told us that Jess was rarely home because he was regularly taking her to doctor's appointments and therapy sessions. Jess's phone was mysteriously always broken, and we could not speak to her directly to verify what she was doing during the day.

Since Aaron's Good Will drop off at our house, Jess has been able to purchase a power wheelchair with her monthly disability money that Aaron so graciously allowed her to receive. Jess has also paid all her accruing medical bills that Aaron did not pay. She has purchased a conversion mobility van. Jess now pays out-of-pocket for her therapy.

Perhaps the saddest thing I have to say about all of this is that the doctor told us that Jessica most likely could have been walking today. That is if Aaron had taken the time and spent the money to get Jessica the medical care she so desperately needed.

No, instead, he told us that the doctors informed him that Jess had gone as far as she was going to go and that he should divorce her so she could go into a nursing home. His reasoning: The divorce would allow Jess to receive both Medicaid and Medicare (because he makes too much money). The skilled nursing facility would be a better place for Jess because she could receive round-the-clock medical care. He would bring Eva to visit her at his leisure. What else?

I can't write any more about him and his reasons for leaving his disabled wife. I might write something I'd regret. I think his actions speak louder than any words I could type.

The divorce is progressing as we expected. At every turn, Jess is consistently asking for what is rightfully hers. He's refusing. Jess has asked for shared custody of Eva. He wants to have Eva more than Jess has her. Jess has asked for her money back so that she can pay her out-of-pocket expenses for her therapy (she didn't qualify for either Medicare or Medicaid at the time).

He's asked that she just forget about the money. She's asked for help with her attorney fees, and he's asked for help with his. She's asked for alimony. He's asked not to pay alimony. He doesn't want to pay child support either, just give Jess half of the money that was already allocated for Eva through Jess's disability. He is currently receiving the money for Eva. And, so it goes.

As of right now, there is no end in sight. His attorney has divorced him because of "irreconcilable differences." How ironic—he hasn't gotten a new one—so, we wait.

Now that Aaron is representing himself, he's started with the texts and emails to me. I try not to answer. I try to remain cool, calm, and collected.

Cool, calm, and collected. I looked it up. That expression was used as a synonym for: "cool as a cucumber" dating to the 1800s. I learned that the insides of cucumbers are approximately 20 degrees cooler than the outside air.

I wish that my insides would remain 20 degrees cooler than the outside air in Florida. I want to cool my insides when Aaron starts blaming Jess and me for this nasty divorce.

His complaints are many, but the most fervid rant is about how Jess must have money to burn (to pay her attorney) and that all I care about is money. Can anyone say "projection" here? Surely, Aaron doesn't care one hoot about money. His other complaint is that Jess is making this divorce so much more difficult than it has to be. No blame-shifting here.

Jess has a mirror image exercise that she does for therapy. She looks at her right hand (the good hand) in the mirror, opening and closing it while her left hand (clenched hand) is behind the mirror. This exercise tricks her brain into thinking that the left hand is doing everything the right hand is doing. I think Aaron should spend less time exercising in front of the mirror at the gym and more time with a mirror image exercise. After he's done admiring himself in the gym mirror, he could do divorce mirror therapy.

Perhaps the cruelest thing he has done is to inform Jess that Eva will be cared for by "responsible adults" over the summer while he is at work. Jess asked Aaron to provide the names of these individuals, and he refused. Jess has told him in writing that she is available and able to care for Eva while he works. Aaron doesn't care. He is in direct violation of the court order giving Jess the right to have her daughter with her when he is unavailable for more than four hours.

So, he has deliberately left Eva in the care of his girlfriend, Dolores, and has made sure that Jess is well aware of the arrangement. He is encouraging Eva to form a bond with Dolores while continuing to minimize Jess's role in her daughter's life. This reality made my blood boil. I guess this whole mess strikes an emotional chord with me that I cannot fully grasp. I imagine that it takes me back to a time when a new mother was pushed into my life, and I was expected to accept and love her. I was only five and didn't understand why my mommy was gone. I certainly couldn't understand why a new mommy was coming into my life.

I feel the same way with Eva, but it's different. Eva has her mommy. I keep telling her that. Her mommy is here, and she doesn't need a new mommy. My feelings are for my daughter, as well as for my granddaughter. I feel compelled to protect both of them. I don't want either of them to hurt the way I hurt.

I want to take Eva and her mother away from all of this. Start over again. Somewhere safe and happy. A beach would be nice. A faraway beach where we could spend our days making drip castles in the sand, and I could impart all my wisdom on my granddaughter as we watch beautiful sunsets over the water. I'm dreaming now. Suddenly, reality hits me hard. It blasts into my subconscious with a thunderous roar, and my reverie is short-lived.

Reflection

I think my inside temperature just increased by at least 20 degrees! I'm no longer "cool as a cucumber." I'm "mad as a hornet" (also from the 1800s). I'm allowing Aaron and Dolores too much leeway into my psyche. Heck, I've given them superhighway access right into my soul.

Time to get off this soul train before it becomes a soul drain. I need to stop writing about the divorce and start writing about something fun.

Chapter 37

UNgraceful

Mar 2017

To give everyone a break from the doldrums, we decided on a road trip to The Villages this past weekend. The Villages is always a fun place to visit. I even wrote a story about a recent visit to The Villages.

Village Idiots

My much older sister Lisa recently moved to The Villages in Ocala, Florida. The Villages is a retirement community for seniors that don't act their age. The residents of this Stepford-like community could have been actors in the movie Cocoon, where the elderly residents of the Sunny Shores retirement home are suddenly rejuvenated by swimming in an alien "life force" pool.

The inhabitants of The Villages drive around in $40,000 souped-up golf carts, play golf, pickleball, swim, and do aerobics by day and party all night (well, maybe until 9 p.m.). I have yet to see one senior with a walker or wheelchair, and I have never seen a cemetery anywhere in The Villages.

I think that the "life force" rejuvenation must be in the piped-in music that's played in the village squares or perhaps it's in the drinking water. I'm just saying...

Anyway, whenever my much older sister and I get together, it seems we always end up in a laughing fit—

often somewhere very public. You would think that in a place like The Villages, there would be a "Depend" factory or something. I mean, the place has three zip codes and only seniors.

However, there is nothing in The Villages that screams "old people live here!" There isn't the slightest hint that women with weak bladders exist in The Villages. But I know this is a falsehood since Lisa does, in fact, live in The Villages. I could also live there despite being much younger than my sister.

I have visited Lisa several times now since her move to Florida. I was almost certain that I would be banned from visiting after the last time. I kept expecting a certified letter from the village police stating that I have proven myself to be unfit for retirement to The Villages due to weak bladder syndrome and some other minor problems that accompany "normal" aging.

I couldn't help the puking in the middle of the street incident (and no, I wasn't drinking). And it wasn't my fault that I didn't know the golf cart tunnel had a speed limit of 5mph, and you're supposed to use your horn and lights, but that's another story.

Since it didn't appear that I had been banned from The Villages, my whole family decided to go to my sister's for Easter. Thirteen people arrived at Lisa's house, and we were all spending the night. After dinner, Lisa asked me to help her get the blow-up mattress into her tiny office and put the sheet on it.

"Sure," I innocently said as I gathered the sheets and blankets and put them in the office while Lisa blew up the mattress in the living room.

"Good God! Is Godzilla going to sleep on that thing?" I asked as I watched the blow-up mattress take on a life of its own.

"How are we supposed to move that into your little office?"

"Oh, you're being melodramatic," Lisa said. "It'll fit just fine."

"Okay," I said as I attempted to grab one end of the mattress, "let's do this."

The mattress was at least a foot thick and appeared to be king size. Grabbing the stupid thing proved to be more of a challenge than I anticipated.

"Why didn't you blow this up in the room?" I asked as we struggled to twist and turn the mattress so it would fit down the hall and through the door.

"I didn't want to wake the baby," my sister whispered as the mattress scraped along the wall right outside the baby's room.

By the time we got it through the door, I was dripping in sweat, and my sister's hair was matted to her forehead. I couldn't help it. I started laughing hysterically and had to wrap my legs in knots.

I quickly let go of the mattress and ducked into the nearby bathroom before the inevitable happened. I'm sure my sister could hear me still laughing in the bathroom.

"What's so funny?" Lisa asked as I returned.

"You should see yourself," I laughed. "Your hair is matted to your forehead, and you're sweating profusely. We haven't even gotten the stupid mattress on the floor yet."

"Well, you don't look too hot yourself," she retorted. "Let's just get this bed made before we wake the baby."

After pushing the furniture aside, we were able to fit the monstrosity in the room—barely. I grabbed the fitted sheet and made a heroic attempt to put one end on the corner of the mattress, where it was wedged in the room. I couldn't get any leverage, so I lay on the mattress and attempted to start at the far corner first.

While I was reaching for the far corner, Lisa got the bright idea to lie across her end of the mattress and attempt to put the sheet on the corner diagonal from me. Unfortunately, when Lisa put weight on the end of the bed, she launched me off the bed—kind of like a mattress bounce-house. I landed under the desk in a laughing fit. Lisa was still lying across the bottom of the bed, panting as if she had just run a marathon, trying desperately to get the sheet to stay.

As I crawled out from under the desk, I had to climb onto the mattress because there was nowhere else for me to go. My weight on the bed caused Lisa to roll off her end, popping the sheet off the corner. At this point, Lisa dashed out of the room in a mad rush, presumably for the bathroom. She left me lying on the bed, laughing my head off with the sheet in a heap next to me.

When she returned, she joined me on the mattress for another feeble attempt at sheet control. Surely, two college graduates should be able to figure out a way to put a fitted sheet on an oversized blow-up mattress. Instead, we were behaving like two village idiots!

Well, after much contemplation, we devised a foolproof plan where each of us, holding one corner of the sheet, would roll from the middle to the ends of the bed. The key to this working was moving in tandem. Then neither of us would reach the edge of the bed before the other, causing roll-off. Sadly, our plan failed miserably, and we both rolled off either end of the bed.

I guess it had been at least 30 minutes by the time the commotion drew the attention of my two daughters. When they entered the office, they found their aunt and mother both lying on the floor out of breath and laughing uncontrollably.

My daughters could have helped. They could have each grabbed a sheet corner. But, no. Instead, they got out their handy dandy cell phones and hit the record button. They even dared to suggest that we had been drinking. As God is my witness, I had nothing to drink that night.

I could continue with this sad story of two desperate women just trying to provide a restful place for their ungrateful children. I could tell you how the ungrateful children stood there recording the scene, never lifting so much as a finger to hook in a sheet corner.

I could tell you how the baby never stirred, nor did any of the sleeping men in the house. I could go on describing how two brave women continued to wrestle the cunning sheet, but, as the saying goes, a picture is worth a thousand words.

Or, in this case, a video is worth a thousand laughs. Oops, the girls erased the pictures and the videos by mistake.

So sad. Anyway, I'm expecting my certified letter from The Villages any day now!

Chapter 38

UNforgettable

June 2017

Indomitable Will

When Aaron dropped Jess off at our home, he told us that Jess had made all the progress she was expected to make; hence it would be perfectly reasonable to place her in a nursing home to live out her days. Of course, we were horrified at the idea of our 30-year-old daughter rotting in a nursing home while Aaron had a grand old time getting on living his life with Dolores.

So, we made arrangements for Jess to receive ongoing intensive therapy in Tampa. The results have been remarkable. Jess has been fitted with a specialized leg brace and walker so that she is now able to walk quite a distance. Her indomitable will is evident in everything she does—especially walking.

Creak, scrape, creak, scrape; the repetitive sound makes its way down the fluorescent-lit hallway as the walker slowly advances over the spit-polished hospital floor. The movement is slow but steady as each step is carefully maneuvered to keep the walker from zigzagging off course.

The final destination is only about 15 feet away, a meandering tortoise might reach the door quicker, but nothing will get in the way of Jess's determination. She WILL walk into this room even if it takes her all day to do it! Creak, scrape, creak, scrape—almost there. The smile on her face belies the struggle it takes to make this journey.

With each creak and scrape, I film the slow progress, and my heart feels as though it might burst with joy. I know this struggle all too well. I know how long it took to get here to this day, this hour...this moment.

Jess's struggle started almost two years ago. No one ever thought that the day would come when she would push her walker down the hall. Certainly, no one thought it would be this soon. Creak, scrape, creak, scrape; her smile lights up her entire face. Jess's aunt is behind her, as always, the ever-present encourager.

On she goes. Her braced leg has a mind of its own; wayward and helter-skelter, it tries to veer off course. Jess doesn't give in—Jess doesn't give up. Jess doesn't allow her impetuous leg to rue the day. This day is extraordinarily special!

The door to his room is just ahead. He doesn't know Jess is coming. If he hears her, he probably suspects it's only one of the many mechanical assistant machines almost everyone in this wing of the hospital uses. He would have no reason to suspect that the person operating the contraption was anyone of any specific interest.

I move to the door of his room. I'm shaking. The tears are flowing now—I can't help it. I'm about to open the door to Gavin's room. Courageous Gavin. Fearless Gavin. Audacious Gavin. Gavin, the brave!

There's no describing Gavin. Like there's no describing Jess. In this cosmos, God found a way to put these two indomitable spirits together. Together, they each faced insurmountable odds, and together, each triumphed.

Gavin was Jess's first-grade student, her favorite (she always reminds me). He was born with Cerebral Palsy and faced many obstacles in his young life. I like to think that Jess was chosen to be Gavin's teacher because of her unique way with children who face challenging situations. I have no doubt that God's mighty hand was at work when Gavin became her special charge.

Although Gavin is now nine, he has kept in touch with Jess over the years. Jess taught with Gavin's grandmother, and he often visited Jess in her room before and after school. When Jess suffered her brain aneurysm, Gavin frequently came to the hospital. He always told me that someday he and Mrs. R would do physical therapy together.

There were days when we had doctors tell us that Jenn's prognosis was very bleak, but Gavin, the brave, would always tell me that Mrs. R was going to get better and would walk again someday. He never wavered in his belief that he would one day walk side by side with his teacher.

Over this past year, Gavin has had some major surgeries. We learned that Gavin was going to St. Joseph's Hospital in Tampa for his most recent surgery. Since Jess goes to Tampa General for her outpatient therapy, I called Gavin's grandma and asked her if we could stop and see Gavin at St. Joseph's on Monday. We were already on the road, and I expected that we could visit Gavin after Jess was done with her therapy.

Imagine my surprise when Gavin's grandma told me that he had been transferred to Tampa General Children's wing for therapy. Jess was so excited to learn that Gavin was right next door to the building where she gets her treatments. Not only that, but Jess had put on her "team Gavin" tee-shirt that morning!

It's a good thing that I called Gavin's grandma on Monday because, in true Gavin fashion, he was already amazing all the doctors at Tampa General with his determination and grit. They were already talking about an early release since Gavin had made such tremendous progress. This last surgery was very serious because it involved his spine. He wasn't expected to walk for at least three weeks. However, the day of his surgery, he stood. The day after his surgery, he walked.

Now, this day, this hour, this moment has come. I open the door. Gavin's face lights up as Jess appears in his doorway. She gradually makes her way step by step into his room. Gavin sits up. Slowly, painfully he moves to place both feet on the floor. Then, taking his father's hand, Gavin stands.

Deliberately, Gavin places one foot in front of the other and haltingly walks over to his teacher. Each of them has walked a path that few of us will ever have the privilege to experience. They have traversed rugged terrain not meant for the faint of heart. Many people grow weary from life's struggles, but Gavin and Jess never become disheartened.

Jess's favorite word is "perfect," and Gavin's favorite saying is, "never give up." They are the perfect never give up team. I've learned from them that facing trials is about the fight in your heart as well as the heart in your fight. As Gandhi so aptly put it: "Strength does not come from physical capacity; it comes from indomitable will."

Chapter 39

UNfair

Kevin

September 2017

I looked up "indomitable will" because I wanted to understand its meaning accurately. The dictionary defines it as "incapable of being subdued or overcome, or courage unconquerable." I need unconquerable courage right now. I need to borrow Jess's indomitable will because I don't think I can go on any longer.

No parent should ever lose a child. Isn't that what they say? Parents are supposed to go before their kids. It doesn't fit the natural order of things for kids to precede their parents in death. In a way, I lost Jessica already. I lost the daughter that was a 29-year-old wife, mother, and teacher. I lost the daughter that was living a full, independent life. I lost the young woman she had become. In some respects, I gained a child back with Jessica. I am thankful that God blessed me with her all over again. Yet, I pray and hope for her full independence once more.

At the same time that Jessica was in the hospital, we were asked if we wanted to take our four-year-old granddaughter, Kevin's daughter, into our home. It seems that neither Kevin nor the mother of his child was able to care for her any longer. Protective Services was trying to place her with family. We couldn't take our granddaughter at that time for obvious reasons, and she was placed with her maternal grandmother.

Kevin was coming to the hospital intermittently to visit Jess, and we begged him to do everything in his power to work hard at getting his daughter back. We offered to help with housing or whatever else he needed. After we talked to him, we didn't see Kevin again for a very long time. My only contact with him was through social networking, which was very sporadic.

Every time I saw Kevin, I would tell him how much I loved and missed him. Every time, he would say to me that he'd do a better job of staying in touch. It never happened. Kevin would return to his world of escape. I believe he just wanted to escape his demons that forever haunted him, and the lure of drugs seduced him to go AWOL from life.

Then, on September 22, Kevin went AWOL from life forever. I learned about his death on social media. RIP was all over his Facebook page. That was it. The police didn't call us or show up at our house. Kevin's "real family" didn't contact us. His "real sister" (the only family contact in his phone under "sis") told the police that she didn't even know if we legally adopted him. Even though he had our last name, they assumed that the family had been contacted since they spoke with his sister.

Finally, after contacting the police, I learned the truth. I learned that Kevin died in his apartment from an overdose of heroin laced with Fentanyl. I discovered that his roommate didn't report his death for over six hours because he thought that Kevin was just passed out on the floor. The police were kind enough to accept that I was indeed his mother and assured me that the only communication would be with me or Kevin's father. Then, they told me that I could go and claim his body at the medical examiner's office.

So, today, I will claim the body of my son.

Last night I dreamt that he was running through a field of wildflowers with his two favorite dogs, Shadow and Toby. In my dream, he was just a boy. In real life, he grew to be a man on the outside, but on the inside, I think he was still that scared little boy who showed up at my home with his caseworker, his brother, his garbage bag full of his belongings and his "life book."

Eight years of "life" were stored in his book—all three pages of it. I wanted so much to fill the rest of his pages with joy and happiness. I wanted to fill them with a "real family" with real parents and real sisters that would love him unconditionally. I wanted so much for him. He was my son, after all. No, he wasn't my birth child, but what does that matter?

Today, I am beating myself up for all the things I didn't say and didn't do. I keep seeing the snapshots in my head that should have been filling up his life book: Kevin hugging his dogs and Mel, our cat. Kevin teaching Lucy how to ride a bike without training wheels when she was just three-years-old. Kevin standing in the water, holding the electric Christmas lights outside and almost electrocuting himself! Kevin sitting with me as I drew him a picture of our family with him and his brother in it.

Twenty years later, when he gave me that picture back for my birthday, I could see where it had been folded and refolded. No doubt, it meant a lot to him. It might have even had a special place in his life book.

I couldn't give him all that he needed, though. I tried. God knows I tried. I never stopped loving my son even after years of separation. I prayed for him. I kept telling him how much I loved him. I wanted to save him from his self-destruction, but I couldn't.

He wrestled his invisible demons alone. I wasn't allowed into the wrestling ring with him, and I couldn't wear his boxing gloves for him. I would have. I keep telling myself that I would have done whatever I could. Did I? Did I do everything I could? I don't know. I do know that this was one battle he had to fight on his own. I could blame myself—I do blame myself.

Perhaps the blame should be laid at the feet of a heartless bureaucratic system that doesn't protect innocent children in foster care. The court system keeps returning these kids to parents that clearly cannot and should not have the privilege of keeping their children. Kevin and his brother had been tossed around from foster home to foster home and back to his "family" time and time again since they were toddlers. His early years were a living hell for him and his brother.

His scars never healed from those early years. He hid them. He buried them, and he allowed them to take hold somewhere in the "not good enough" part of his being. He took himself and his scars to the dark side. He may have allowed his body to visit the dark side, yet there was a bright side to Kevin as well.

I think, in the end, the bright side won. I have to believe that. Kevin was a kind person. I remember one time we were in the Smoky Mountains visiting my friend, Carol. Carol is like a grandmother to my kids. Carol loves hummingbirds. I'll never forget how excited Kevin was when he found a hummingbird feeder that he just had to give to Grandma Carol. It was so important to him to make sure she got the feeder. He was so excited to send Carol that feeder. Carol reminded me just the other day that she still has her hummingbird feeder. After all these years, she still treasures it.

Kevin was the kind of kid and man that would do anything for anybody. That's how I want to remember him. I want to remember the boy and his dogs— carefree. Is there such a thing as being free of care? I think that is where he is now. He's somewhere where he doesn't have to care anymore about being good enough. He's somewhere where he can run free with his beloved pets, where he is not running from or to anything.

I want to believe that he is home. He is in a place where love is unconditional. He is in a home where he doesn't have to drag a garbage bag behind him or carry a book of memories. He is in a home where the only comfort he needs are loving arms that will forever surround him and never judge him. Today, I will claim the body of my son, but Jesus has claimed his soul. For that, I am forever grateful.

Chapter 40

UNfinished

The Now

The truth is life will go on. This story could have no ending because it will continue well past my obituary. However, for the sake of stopping somewhere, now seems like an excellent place to end. It's the beginning of the end—now. Now, in terms of time, is the only place that matters. Now is all we have. We don't know if tomorrow will ever come. Yesterday is only a fleeting memory—or in Jess's case, not a memory at all.

So, here I type in the "now." All I can say about now is that we have made it this far and are hopeful that tomorrow will bring more "nows." Yesterday was Jess's birthday, and she had an appointment with her surgeon for a check-up. She could have been upset that she had to spend her birthday at the doctor's office. However, instead of being upset, she said she was happy to have the opportunity to thank the man that gave her one more birthday.

Jess knows all about "now" because that truly is all she has. She won't remember today that she went to see her surgeon yesterday (unless I remind her). She'll get out of bed this morning and ask me, "What are we doing today?" I've told her at least three times last night what we are doing today. She'll go to school and volunteer, teaching kids how to read, yet she won't be able to remember when we get out of the car at home that she was just at her beloved school where she used to teach first grade.

Is this sad? I don't know. It's just what we deal with now. When now is all you have, there's something you learn. You learn that every second of every day is valuable. You learn to fill those seconds with humor and love. You learn that a kiss is not just a kiss; it could be the last. You learn that words matter a lot. You learn that people matter a lot. Now makes you think about why you do what you do. It puts things into perspective. When now is all you have, you cannot worry about the future or dwell on the past.

"There's always tomorrow" is a falsehood. There isn't always tomorrow. That's the truth. So, I wonder what I should do with now. Should I spend my now spewing Yiddish curses at Aaron? Should I fill my now with anger or worry? Should I allow someone else's now to creep into my psyche and poison it? No, I shouldn't, but I often do. I know that I have to become more like Jess and fill my now with joy—whatever it takes.

Last night, I was tucking Eva into bed. We always go through a routine of "butterfly kisses" with our eyelashes. Eva expanded our routine to include Eskimos kisses, chin kisses, ear kisses, hair kisses, and cheek kisses. Sometimes we add elbows and hands, or whatever else we think of. Last night, Eva asked me to give her a necklace kiss. At first, I wasn't sure what she was referring to. Then, I realized she was talking about my grandmother's cross that I always wear.

"Nana," Eva said, "I want to kiss the cross goodnight so that my kiss stays close to your heart all night."

This is what living in the moment is all about. It's about those moments when life pierces through the outer barrier right into your soul. It's those moments that make us cry and laugh and feel deeply. I felt so blessed to share that moment with my little granddaughter. I told her that my cross would one day be close to her heart to remind her that, even when I go to be with Jesus, I will always be in her heart like my grandma is in my heart right now.

So, I'm typing now. I'm writing now. I'm looking at my donkeys out the window now. I'm listening to the rooster crowing now. I'm living in the moment for now. It's nice and peaceful. I'm waiting for Jess's voice to call, "I'm ready to get up now." That's it. No worries.

I may be a drama momma sometimes. I may visit the Land of UN more often than I'd like. However, it is my solemn vow that I will try to live in now and leave the drama to another momma. Perhaps Aaron's momma, Anne, will pick up the mantle.

Epilogue 2018

One Year Later

The final trial for the divorce has concluded, and Jess has emerged victorious. As the judge quickly surmised from Aaron's self-defense prior to the final trial: "He looks with his eyes, listens with his ears, and understands like a wall." Perhaps the judge also realized that there was no furniture in Aaron's attic. I could add a few more Yiddish sayings: "Empty barrels make the most noise." or "You'll see it when you see your own ears."

Aaron didn't see any of his wrongdoing. He finally hired another attorney to represent him in the final divorce trial. His new attorney had been arrested for DUI, and her mugshot was being handed out in front of the courthouse by the arresting officer. The officer wanted to make a point about how corrupt the court system is in this county. I cannot make this stuff up!

Before the trial even began, the judge ordered both attorneys into his chambers and announced that he would be awarding lifetime alimony to Jess. He also informed them that Aaron would pay all of Jess's back medical bills and her attorney's fees. The judge told them that the parties would continue with shared custody and shared decision making for the minor child. He said that his order awarding school decisions for the minor child to Jessica stands.

The judge admonished Aaron's attorney for wasting his time by allowing this to go to trial. He told both attorneys to work everything out with each of their clients and return to him with a proposal.

The final proposal contained all of the judge's suggestions and included a time-sharing agreement for Eva. It was everything Jessica wanted. Aaron turned to his mommy and said, "I'm screwed for life!"

At the trial's conclusion, Jessica got up and grabbed her walker and began her exit from the courtroom. She made her deliberate passage down the aisle with the attorneys, the court staff, Aaron, Aaron's mom, aunt, and our family watching her slow descent.

"Jessica, I am so proud of you," announced Jess's attorney. "You are amazing and have come so far since our first meeting."

"I'm so proud of her, too," said Aaron's mom. "I ask about her every day."

"It's amazing what therapy can do for someone," replied Aaron's aunt.

Not being one to keep my mouth shut, I made a statement to the entire courtroom. "This past year for Jess sure as hell beat sitting in a nursing home," I said. "Oh, excuse me, I mean 'a skilled nursing facility'!"

The End

Contact Page

Drama Momma in the Land of UN is available on
Amazon.com in paperback and Kindle versions.

If you would like to contact Gwen Thorne,
please use the following:

gwenthorne01@gmail.com

Made in the USA
Columbia, SC
19 March 2020